Defending the Body
Unraveling the Mysteries of Immunology

DEFENDING THE BODY

Unraveling the Mysteries of Immunology

JOEL DAVIS

Atheneum
New York
1989

LP

Atheneum
Macmillan Publishing Company
866 Third Avenue, New York, N.Y. 10022
Collier Macmillan Canada, Inc.

Library of Congress Cataloging-in-Publication Data
Davis, Joel, ——
    Defending the body : unraveling the mysteries of immunology / Joel Davis.
        p.   cm.
    Includes index.
    ISBN 0-689-11946-1
    1. Immunology—Popular works. 2. Immunology—Research—Popular works. I. Title.
QR181.7.D38 1989
616.07'9—dc19   88-32162
                                                      CIP

Macmillan books are available at special discounts for bulk purchases for sales promotions, premiums, fund-raising, or educational use. For details, contact:
    Special Sales Director
    Macmillan Publishing Company
    866 Third Avenue
    New York, N.Y. 10022

10 9 8 7 6 5 4 3 2 1

Printed in the United States of America

10-16-89

To
JULIANA MOON
JOHN STURGEON
PEGGIE WOLFSON
in memoriam

---

*and to the men and women
around the world who have dedicated their lives
to defending the body against disease*

Contents

Preface

During the eighteen months I spent working on the book you hold in your hand, I learned (or relearned) some fascinating things about scientists. One such lesson was that many researchers feel they must be careful in their conversation with journalists, reporters, science writers. Several people politely declined to be interviewed, and I respect that decision. Especially in the case of scientists working for corporations, the reasons for reticence are understandable: The competition is lurking everywhere, secrets to steal. The rules of behavior for corporate scientists are almost the same as those for academic scientists—almost, but not quite. Then there's the matter of *competence*. Does this guy really know what I'm talking about? And finally there's the matter of—oh, how to put it?—let's call it "the simplifying instinct." Talk to a group of scientists (from any discipline—it doesn't matter if they're astronomers, immunologists, or desert botanists) about reporters, and they'll tell you horror stories. Misperceptions! they will cry aloud. Misquotations! Outright lies! Reporters are devious, unscrupulous, looking only for a "hot" story or a "sexy" quote. And for headlines. They never get the facts right.

A friend and colleague of mine had run into this problem while writing a book on medicine. He had talked with a prominent researcher, and the interview had not gone very well. Later, the man was apparently not pleased with the way he was portrayed in the book. "So for God's sake," my friend later warned me, "if you ever interview this fellow for *your* book, don't tell him you know me." As it turned out, I did interview the same man, and my talk with him was friendly and fruitful. Perhaps it was a matter of personalities; perhaps it was because I didn't mention his name; perhaps the researcher was in a bad mood when my colleague talked with him, or in a good mood when I did.

Or perhaps it was because the agenda of the science writer is never quite the same as that of the scientist. Truth is sometimes a slippery fellow. Any theologian or biblical scholar will tell you that a lot gets lost in translation from original language to current patois. To report in pure scientific language the results of an experiment would probably be utterly baffling gobbledygook to any average reader of any average newspaper or magazine. Finding accurate synonyms for some scientific nomenclature is oftimes an impossible task. The reporter resorts to whatever seems to work. A science writer, who specializes in reporting the interesting breakthroughs (and sometimes boring minutiae) of some discipline, usually tries harder than the general assignment reporter to come up with a reasonably accurate translation. Some scientists—astronomer Carl Sagan comes to mind, as do physician Lewis Thomas and molecular biologist Lee Hood—are genuinely interested in conveying the importance and excitement of their work to the general public. They take the time to educate the reporter (and the science writer, who may not always be a scientist), to rephrase statements, to reprove, correct, and help in the translation. It is unfortunate that there are few Carl Sagans and Lewis Thomases in science.

I also relearned the difference between how we *think* scientists work, and how it really is. Real life is rarely straightforward or linear, and few of us hear background music when we accomplish something notable. Yet it often seems that scientific advances are portrayed as happening in this fashion, with the great breakthroughs accompanied by flashes of lightning and blares of trumpets. The average person on the street comes away from such an account (usually encapsulated in a forty-five second report on the evening television news or a 400-word newspaper column, less often in a 2,500-word magazine article) feeling that "doing science" has little relation to everyday life.

The truth, of course, is that "doing science" is often as winding a road as "doing art," "doing theology," or even "doing plumbing." Like any other human endeavor, science has its highs. They come rarely. Doing science is mostly a lot of hard work, long days, months, and years of frequent tedium sprinkled with the frustrations of missed insights and dead ends. But every scientist worth his or her salt lives in anticipation of that intellectual high that happens when something truly *new* is found for the first time. My interviews with the people you will meet in this book gave me a much clearer insight into how the science of immunology has moved forward in the last several years and how it continues to move. It is being moved with hard work. And the people doing the moving are themselves driven by impulses common to us all: the desire to know more, to stretch themselves a bit. Sometimes, there is the high.

In this regard, I did learn something that many readers will find surprising. Most of the major figures in the explosion of immune-system research—whether they are publicly prominent or quietly behind the scenes—rarely if ever spend time working at the laboratory bench. Like it or not, they are in the management business. That, however, doesn't diminish the importance of their contribution to the advancement of immunology. Most of them are in their midthirties to midforties, and at the peak of their energies. Robert Kamen, John Farrar, Leroy Hood, and the others I met are people who harness their drive for excellence to their immense creativity. Their work is changing the face of immunology.

The extent to which I have succeeded in portraying some of those who are defending the body is due in very large part to the kind help and assistance I received from many people. My thanks to Hardy Chan, Daniel Drachman, William Earnshaw, John Farrar, Donald Francis, L. Patrick Gage, Leroy Hood, Robert Kamen, Ronald Levy, Barbara Nepom, Gerald Nepom, Enzo Paoletti, Robert Schwartz, Linda Sheperd, Elaine Kinney Thomas, Richard Thorne, Irving Weisman, Lennart Wetterberg, and Tom White. To those whose names I have inadvertently omitted, my apologies. Not all the comments of all these people ended up in the final version of this book, but they were all generous with their time and knowledge. Any errors of fact are mine.

My thanks also to my parents, Gerald and Toni Davis; my editors at Atheneum, Lawrence McIntyre and Margaret Talcott; my agent, Russell Galen; and Kerry Beaulieu, Bed & Breakfast USA, Ltd., Frank and Cindy Catalano, Marie Celestre, Jack Christensen, Judy Flinders, David Gerardot, Perle Goodwin, Armando Guzman, Dick and Linda Hancock, Mary Krauss, Jay and Susan Lerman, Suzanne Loebl, Avrill Logan, the Olympia (Washington)

AIDS Task Force, Michael J. Ryan, Saint Michael's Catholic Church (Olympia, Washington), the San Francisco AIDS vigilers, Nancy Sigafoos and Dorothy Tenkhoff, and Joy Yancey.

And to "the Wind that blows where it will": thank you for blowing my way.

Defending the Body
Unraveling the Mysteries of Immunology

1 Breaking the Code

On November 20, 1987, Leroy Hood received the Lasker Award in ceremonies at Rockefeller University in New York City. Hood, the chairman of the Biology Division at the California Institute of Technology in Pasadena, California, shared the Lasker with three other researchers in immunology, including Susumu Tonegawa of MIT and Philip Leder of Harvard. Hood, Leder, and Tonegawa received the award for their work in unraveling one of the most mysterious yet important secrets of the immune system. They had led three separate research teams at three separate institutions in a successful search for the answer to the question that lies at the core of immunology: How does the immune system defend the body against *nearly everything* the universe can throw at it?

Immunology is the medical science which studies the immune system, that marvelously complex network of cells and chemicals that keeps us healthy most of the time,

1

and which usually cures us when we fall ill. In essence, this elaborate system is able to recognize that a particular substance is Not-Self: that it is a foreigner, an invader, or a turncoat such as a cancerous cell. By checking certain features of molecules on the surfaces of cells, viruses, or other microscopic objects, the immune system's components identify those molecules that are not part of the body.

This immunological power of recognition is not all that different from, say, telling a real peach from a wax peach. Suppose someone presents you with two objects that look like peaches. You soon know that one is not a real peach. Its skin—its "surface feature"—doesn't feel right. It is not fuzzy. It is smooth and waxy. It is, in fact, a wax peach. What's more, you will now *remember* what that wax peach feels like. Later, even years later, you will be able in an instant to identify an object as a wax peach and not the real thing. The biological process of recognizing, selectively eliminating, and remembering the shape and feel of foreign invaders and harmful cells is called the *immune response*. The immune system acts, in a remarkable sense, like the brain. In order to defend the body, it works to identify, act upon, and remember foreign substances. Exactly how the immune system does this had puzzled researchers for decades. Hood, Leder, and Tonegawa cracked the code.

The Lasker was not the first award Hood had received in his more than twenty years as a practicing molecular biologist. It would probably not be his last. But it was far and away the most prestigious award he had yet received. Perhaps the only honor for work in biology or medicine more eminent than the Lasker is the Nobel Prize in Physiology or Medicine. Those who pay attention to these things (and there are more than a few who do) ventured the confident prediction that Hood would also add that one to his trophy case in 1987.

As it turned out, Susumu Tonegawa alone received the Nobel Prize in Physiology or Medicine in 1987. Leder and Hood, though, bore no grudges, freely acknowledging that Tonegawa richly deserved the Nobel medal and money. For Hood, at least, awards are not nearly as important or as satisfying as the search itself. He always seems to have four or five different projects in the works at once, with different teams of Cal Tech students busy in his laboratory, puzzling out some new mystery. This driving, charging manner, this constant search for new challenges and questions to answer, is not out of character for a man who often spends his vacations climbing mountains.

There are plenty of questions for Hood and his colleagues to answer. Indeed, medical work related to immunology or the immune system has long been a good ticket to fame, if not fortune. The very first Nobel Prize for Physiology or Medicine, awarded in 1901, went to the German physician Emil Adolf von Behring for demonstrating a way to immunize people against diphtheria and tetanus. In 1905 Robert Koch was awarded a Nobel Prize for developing a test for tuberculosis, but he is equally famous for identifying the microscopic organisms that cause TB, cholera, and anthrax. The French physician Charles Laveran received his Nobel Prize in 1907 for work showing how some microscopic creatures called protozoans cause disease. The following year another French researcher, Élie Metchnikoff, shared the medical Nobel with the German physician Paul Ehrlich. Both got the prize for work related to immunology and the immune system. Twenty-five years earlier, Metchnikoff had suggested that certain cells in the bloodstream performed a vital function in protecting the body against foreign invaders. He called them *phagocytes,* or "cell eaters," and they are perhaps better known as "white blood cells." Metchnikoff thought they ate and thus destroyed invading bacteria. Meanwhile, Paul Ehrlich (who's more famous for developing a way to treat syphilis) and the Austrian-born American research Karl Landsteiner were busy demonstrating the importance of other substances to immunity. They called them antibodies.

Landsteiner's and Erhlich's work dominated the still-nascent field of immunology at the beginning of the twentieth century. More than seventy years later, the work of Hood, Tonegawa, and Leder was in the vanguard of immunology. But to appreciate the real importance of what they and others were doing in the mid to late 1970s, it is important to understand how life reproduces itself and how it allows for changes to occur. This is the work of DNA, genes, and chromosomes.

DNA, deoxyribonucleic acid, is literally the building block of life. This elegant molecule on first glance consists of two linear strands joined together by chemical "rungs." It twists around itself in a double helix shape. On closer inspection, DNA is seen to be made of millions of tiny units called *nucleotides.* Each nucleotide is made of two parts: a flattened chemical structure called a base, and a piece of the backbone structure. The latter is made of alternating molecules of sugar and phosphate. The bases stick out of the backbone, connecting together to form the rungs, which join the two sugar phosphate strands together. The bases in DNA come in four varieties, the chemicals adenine, cytosine, guanine, and thymine. They are usually abbreviated as A, C, G, and T. Because of their chemical nature, A only connects to T, and C only connects to G (and, of course, vice versa). If one strand of DNA has an A molecule at one point, the other strand *must* have a T. The same is true when one strand has a G; the opposite strand *must* have a C in the corresponding position. Only when the two bases are properly paired will the two strands of DNA connect together. This is called *complementary base pairing.* This pairing of bases is the key to DNA's retention and transmission of information.

A *chromosome* is a structure inside the nucleus of a cell containing an incredibly long strand of DNA, along with various proteins needed to organize and compact the DNA molecule. Chromosomes come in pairs inside a cell. When the cell divides and multiplies, the chromosome pairs split apart, one to each new daughter cell. Each single chromosome soon creates its double, leaving the new daughter cells with the same number of chromosomes as the parent cell. The process is called *mitosis.*

A *gene* is part of a chromosome. To be precise, it is a small section of DNA containing information for the construction of a protein molecule. So, in the end, DNA is simply a molecule containing information on how to make other molecules—amino acids and proteins, specifically. Genes are those segments of DNA with instructions for a specific protein.

Chromosomes are collections of genes along a strand of DNA. Different species of animals and plants have different numbers of chromosome pairs. Humans have forty-six chromosomes in twenty-three pairs, numbered (and named) 1 through 22 plus X and Y. Twenty-two of them are *somatic* or *autosomal* chromosomes. Both words come from *soma,* the Greek word for "body." The X and Y chromosomes (so-called because under the microscope they look like an X and a Y) are called the sex chromosomes, and carry the code for determining gender and various sex-linked characteristics. The twenty-three pairs of chromosomes contain within them the genetic code for the human body—skin, liver, heart, brain, muscle, bone, gender, eye color, hair color, numbers of fingers and toes—and the immune system.

DNA is Nature's way of creating proteins, and genes and chromosomes are the "books" and "encyclopedias" that contain that DNA information. All proteins are made of combinations of the smaller molecular units called amino acids. About twenty amino acids exist in nature, and every protein that exists, or can ever exist, is made of some combination of amino acids. Proteins range in size from a few dozen to several thousands of amino acids, all arranged in a complex three-dimensional structure.

The method by which genes carry the information to create amino acids and proteins is simplicity itself. It's all in the sequence of As, Ts, Cs, and Gs along the DNA double helix. DNA has an alphabet with just four letters. But these four DNA letters combined in triplet sequences called *codons,* are more than enough to spell out enough genetic words and sentences to create the proteins needed to create a unique human individual.

Some genes carry the instructions to make a molecule similar to DNA, called RNA (ribonucleic acid). RNA is a postcard, if you will, that carries a duplicate of the information in a specific gene. Like DNA, RNA is a double helix molecule. It too has an alphabet of four letters or bases: adenine (A), cytosine (C), guanine (G), and uracil (U). Each of the twenty amino acids is represented by one to six RNA codons. One codon, AUG, codes for the amino acid methionine, for example. The codon UUG spells out the instructions to make the amino acid tryptophan. There is a difference of just one letter between the two. There are two different codons that spell out the code for tyrosine. Any of four codons will produce the amino acid alanine. And serine can be coded for by any of six different codons. Finally, a few codons act as "start" or "stop" signals for the construction of an amino acid or protein. Messenger RNA (or mRNA) carries the gene's codon-encoded information from the DNA in the nucleus to another structure in the cell called a *ribosome.* Ribosomes are the "workbenches" of a cell. Here the information from the DNA, via the mRNA, is translated into amino acids, which a form of RNA called transfer RNA (or tRNA) links together into a protein. The entire process is called *gene expression*.

The transmission of information from DNA to RNA to complete protein is not perfect. Mistakes occasionally occur, called *mutations*. This causes the wrong amino acid to be placed into a particular protein. If a mutation eliminated the A in AUG and inserted a U, the resulting amino acid would not be methionine, but tryptophan. Such a change could be disastrous if the protein in question is, for example, one that affects the development of the fetal brain. On the other hand, if the codon GCA mutates into GCG, the result will still be the amino acid alanine. Nature uses backups, and it pays off by reducing the possibility of mutation damage. Mutations can take place for any of a number of reasons. Some chemicals are mutagenic, causing changes in the DNA messages. Ionizing radiation, such as gamma rays or X rays, also damage the DNA structure and cause mutations. Finally, some mutations simply occur because of imprecise copying of data from DNA to mRNA, or from imperfect copying of data from mRNA to amino acids and proteins in the ribosomes of a cell. Most mutations are damaging—some even lethal. A smaller number may be of no consequence. Every once in a great while, a mutation may end up being useful to the creature in which it occurs.

When the mutation takes place in a creature's somatic cell, it is called a somatic mutation. The consequences of such mutations are limited only to the creature in which it takes place. If the mutation occurs in a germ cell—a sperm or egg cell—it will be passed on to the following generations. If it's a lethal mutation, the child may well die before birth, or never reach reproductive age. If the mutation is innocuous or beneficial, then the child may end up passing it on to *its* descendants. Given plenty of time—say, millions or even billions of years—and plenty of reproductions, mutations become a driving force for change in life forms. Thus a simple code of four letters can be powerful enough to transmit enormously complex forms of information from one creature to its descendants, and at the same time be flexible enough to allow for possibly helpful modifications in that information.

The immune system is a product of DNA. The codes that create our defense network against germs and viruses are carried in our genes and chromosomes. Chromosomes 6 and 14, in particular, are important centers of information for creating the immune system. It is a remarkably powerful and flexible information network, and it has fascinated Leroy Hood for more than a quarter of a century.

Lee Hood is not an immunologist by formal profession. He's a molecular biologist and medical doctor. His interest in immunology stretches back to his days at Johns Hopkins University in the early 1960s, where he got his M.D. The roots stretch down even deeper, though. Hood's scientific interests began in Montana and not with biology but geology.

One warm winter morning in Pasadena, California, I sat in Hood's office in the Braun Building at Cal Tech. The table between us held a bronze-looking abstract sculpture, and piles of books, journals, and papers. There was barely enough room for my tape recorder. We talked about his journey into immunology. It began, he recalled, in Montana, where he was born and raised. His father worked as an electrical engineer for Mountain Bell Telephone Company. After moving about Montana for several years, the family finally settled in Shelby, about thirty-five miles from the Canadian border. "I think those were among the happiest times of my life," he said. "I was doing so many things, and enjoying them all. I was the quarterback for the football team"—which went undefeated in his last three years at Shelby High—"I acted in plays, I edited my high school yearbook; it was exhilarating."

Hood's interest in science started with geology, he recalled, hanging out during high school summer vacations with some geologists who were working at his grandfather's ranch. That he ended up becoming a gene hound rather than a rock hound was due in large part to his high school science teacher. Hood said, "The guy was pretty strong in geology and the natural sciences, but not so strong on the biological sciences. Well, I wanted to learn more, so he encouraged me to learn on my own. I was reading *Science* and *Nature* magazines in high school. It was wonderful!" In fact, Hood had a good enough grasp of biology that he sometimes ended up teaching classes himself. Perhaps it was not too surprising that Hood decided to go to college at the California Institution of Technology, one of this country's greatest centers of learning. Four years later, armed with a degree in biology but wanting much more than what even Cal Tech had given him, Hood headed east, to Baltimore and Johns Hopkins University. His journey into the science of immunology was about to begin in earnest.

Immunology is not a simple discipline, with a few names to memorize and laws to learn. It's as complex as the organic system it studies. Nevertheless, it's possible to sketch out the basic components of the immune system. All living organisms have some sort of defense mechanism against outside invaders like bacteria. First and most basic are the straightforward barriers, "passive" defenses like the skin and mucous membranes and various chemicals in tears, saliva, and sweat. Second, there is a set of chemical compounds called *complement,* which work as "triggers" for other parts of the immune system.

Then there are the more adaptive defenses against invading bacteria and viruses. Metchnikoff's phagocytes are among them. So are the antibodies of Ehrlich and Landsteiner. It didn't seem likely to scientists at the time that two different immunity mechanisms could exist at the same time. In fact, the famous playwright George Bernard Shaw is supposed to have ridiculed Metchnikoff for his "biological romances." But Shaw was wrong, and Metchnikoff was right. And so were Ehrlich and Landsteiner, for that matter. The immune systems of all vertebrate animals have active mechanisms to combat foreign cells or mutated body cells. In all, the immune system has three major sets of soldiers or cells: *B lymphocytes* or B cells, *T lymphocytes* (commonly called T cells), and the phagocytes. Each group of cells is responsible for specific immune activities, but they all interact with one another, with complement, and even with the skin and other parts of the "passive" defenses. The immune system is a kind of democracy with a trillion members, 1 percent of the body's hundred trillion cells. When everything's working correctly, it mounts a tightly coordinated defense force against the body's invaders.

Phagocytes are also called accessory cells, and they are very ancient, evolutionarily speaking. They are even found in sponges, which themselves have only three kinds of cells in all. Phagocytes are primarily responsible for attacking and destroying chemical toxins and substances like asbestos and smoke particles. One kind of accessory cells are the *macrophages.* "Macrophage" means "big eater," and they are. Macrophages are the first line of active defense. They are, in fact, the trigger for the cellular and humoral immune responses. Other accessory cells include *granulocytes* (or neutrophils), *monocytes,* and *eosinophils.*

The other two kinds of immunological soldiers, the T and B lymphocytes, are the repositories of *specific immunity*. That's the ability of the body to recognize a specific foreign substance as Not-Self and to respond appropriately to that specific invader. Some lymphocytes have "memory": they make possible a long-lived immunity to infections like measles, chicken pox, and diphtheria.

The T cells are active soldiers in the immune response. They, along with B cells and phagocytes, arise from precursor cells created in bone marrow. These precursors are called *pluripotent stem cells*. They're "pluripotent" because they seem to have the potential of becoming any of the several kinds of lymphocytes. They're "stem cells" because that's the kind of bone marrow cell they are. T cell precursors undergo a further maturation process in the body's thymus gland, which in childhood (it later shrinks and virtually disappears) is located in the chest cavity near the lungs. Thymus is where the *T* in "T cell" comes from. T cells recognize and directly attack foreign-looking molecules found on fungi, virus-infected cells, and on transplanted foreign cells. T cells also create and release substances called *lymphokines*. These proteins act along with T cells and other immune cells to enhance and modulate the immune response.

T cells come in at least three different varieties or subsets. They include cytotoxic or killer T cells, helper T cells, and suppressor T cells. Cytotoxic Ts, for example, act to kill foreign cells as well as body cells that have been transformed by invading viruses. Cytotoxic Ts are responsible for tissue rejection in organ transplants, for example. They also attack and kill cells in cold sores that have been infected by herpesvirus. Helper Ts do just that—they assist other T cells and B cells in carrying out their role in the immune response. Suppressor Ts act to shut down the immune response when it has accomplished its task of defeating the foreign invaders. T cell actions and reactions are also known as the *cellular immune response.*

The B cells produce the Y-shaped molecules called *antibodies,* which carry out the task of recognizing Not-Self invaders. These are the molecules first identified by Ehrlich and Landsteiner. The substances that antibodies discern are called *antigens* (from the Greek *anti-,* "against," and *genes,* "born"). An antigen may be a substance entering the body from outside: a bacterium, a virus, a toxin, a tiny particle of dust—all can be antigens. Antigens may also be substances within the body itself. Ordinarily the immune system will not make antibodies against the body's own tissues and fluids. But it does happen, for various reasons, and the result is an autoimmune disease like myasthenia gravis or juvenile rheumatoid arthritis.

When the immune system responds to an antigen, the antibodies it produces are not against the entire object. They recognize and respond to small molecular patterns on the surface of the antigen called an *antigenic determinant.* An antigen, like a leopard, has spots all over its coat. Each spot is an antigenic determinant. When an antibody identifies it as a pattern that is Not-Self, the immune system response is triggered. The ultimate result is the destruction of the antigen and the creation of a memory. Like the nervous system, the immune system has a kind of memory called immunologic memory. If the same antigen ever appears again in the body, the immune system will recognize it almost instantly and very rapidly leap to defend the body against it.

B cells are called B because they were first studied in detail in the bursa organ of chickens. Besides triggering various immune mechanisms that kill bacteria, other microbes, and cancer cells, antibodies also neutralize viruses and poisons. B cells and their antibodies make up the *humoral immune response,* so-called because antibodies are carried in the body's fluids and secretions. (The word "humoral" comes from the Latin word *humor* or fluid.) Antibodies are proteins called immunoglobulins, and there are five general classes of them. Within these five classes, though, each antibody is unique, and the immune system's B cells can and do produce a specific antibody for each specific *antigen,* or invading foreign molecule.

Ehrlich and Landsteiner had demonstrated the importance of antibodies in immunity at the beginning of the twentieth century. Nearly three quarters of a century later, Leroy Hood's mentor, William Dreyer, would offer a theoretical explanation of how antibodies worked. Hood himself would later demonstrate the validity of Dreyer's theory.

The first steps toward that moment in Hood's life began at Johns Hopkins University. "I went to medical school not because I wanted to be a physician," Hood said, "but because I was interested in human biology, and I didn't get much of that here at Cal Tech. Then, during my first year at Johns Hopkins, I gave a report on theories of antibody diversity for a microbiology course. Putting together that report convinced me that here was an area of enormous excitement and potential for the future."

Hood was twenty-two at the time, young and open to new ideas and approaches. When he finished medical school, he worked for three years at the National Institutes of Health, and then returned to Cal Tech to get his Ph.D. in biochemistry. He worked on the structure of antibody molecules, in the laboratory of the legendary immunologist William Dreyer.

"Dreyer is really the father of modern molecular immunology," Hood exclaimed. "There is no question about it. If there is one fundamental concept which really illuminated the field, it was *his* insight in 1965. During my graduate work and my three years at the National Institutes of Health, and my first few years here at Cal Tech, I worked at the protein level, analyzing the problem of antibody diversity, trying to differentiate between the two major theories that were then prevalent."

On the one hand, Hood noted, was the argument that there were very few genes that coded for antibody molecules. All of the amazing diversity of antibodies—a unique antibody molecule for recognizing *each* foreign invader or antigen—was generated by *somatic mutation,* mutations happening in the DNA of nonreproductive cells of the body. On the other hand, there was the point of view that Hood liked: There were many antibody genes, and antibody diversity was generated by scrambling and rearranging all these different gene elements.

Partially on the basis of the work done by graduate student Hood, Dreyer in 1965 annunciated a new theory, his "two gene one polypeptide" chain concept of antibody diversity. (A polypeptide is a small protein molecule.) According to this theory, there were indeed only a relatively few genes, or gene fragments, that code for the proteins that make up antibodies. Furthermore, these genes are separated from one another in the chromosome, and come together and combine to form a complete antibody gene. Thus, "two genes equal one polypeptide" or antibody protein.

Hood leaned back and grinned. "Well, what turned out to be the truth is—everybody's right. I mean, it was a theory that had a number of main alternative points of view, and virtually all the points of view have turned out to be central to how you generate antibody diversity." But the truth of Dreyer's theory was not shown until the 1970s.

"Around 1974," said Hood, "it became obvious to me

that you couldn't answer the fundamental questions that needed to be answered about antibody diversity by continuing to be a protein chemist. We had to get down to the molecular level. It was then that Phil Early, a graduate student of mine, agreed to try and learn molecular biology with me. So he set it up in the laboratory. Somewhat later Mark Davis came into the lab as a grad student who was going to work in this area. And those two guys were really the principal architects in all the subsequent work that followed. It took us several years to learn how to do molecular biology, but in the late '70s and early '80s everything came to fruition."

As is often the case in science, the same approach was taking place simultaneously in several other laboratories. Susumu Tonegawa's lab in Switzerland made major contributions to deciphering antibody diversity. So did Phil Leder's lab at MIT. Along with Hood's lab at Cal Tech, they were the three central labs that played a major role in generating and proving the new ideas about antibody diversity. Tonegawa was the real pioneer in using recombinant DNA techniques in this area. He was, in fact, the first one to show formally what Bill Dreyer had hypothesized almost fifteen years earlier; that there were two genes; that they rearranged themselves during the differentiation (that is, the growth and maturing) of B cells; and it was this rearrangement that made it possible for a hundred or so antibody genes to create an entire galaxy of antibody molecules.

Why, exactly, was this breakthrough a breakthrough? Simply put, it was a marvelous answer to a deceptively simple but difficult question: "How does the immune system do what it does?" Several generations of doctors and biologists had puzzled over this question, which is actually at least three questions. First: how can the immune system almost immediately recognize as foreign a substance or object *which it has never before encountered*? Indeed, how can it identify as Not-Self a substance *never before encountered by any living creature that ever existed*? This is the crucial question of "antibody diversity." Second, once that chemical, virus, or bacterium has been tagged as an unfriendly intruder, how does the immune system defend the body against it—and do so without any "slopover" damage to innocent cells? And finally, how does the immune system *remember* the existence of the intruder, so it can quickly attack and destroy any further identical ones?

Lee Hood himself remains awed by the immune system's power. "You know," he told me that winter day in his office, "you and I could walk from here over to my lab, and I could use some machines we have to synthesize an entirely new chemical compound. Something that has never existed before on the face of the earth. I could inject it into you," he continued, "and you know what? Your body would soon make the specific antibody needed to attack and destroy that compound. Even though it has never seen it before. Even though *no living creature has ever seen it before that moment*. But your immune system would quickly make an antibody against it and defeat it. And then remember it for the future." He leaned back in his chair and smiled. "Now—isn't that just *amazing*?"

Hood's work on the genetic basis of antibody diversity was firmly grounded on the bedrock of other information about antibodies. Twenty years earlier other researchers had shown that antibody molecules were made of two kinds of protein chains. They are called "light" and "heavy" chains. The heavy chains are somewhat larger than the light chains, thus the names. An antibody is a molecule made of four chains, two identical heavy chains, and two identical light chains. Sulphide molecules (often called sulphide bridges) hold the two heavy chains together. The heavy chains bend away from each other at one end, forming a Y shape. The light chains, much shorter than the heavy chains, connect via sulphide bridges to the two spread-apart arms of the heavy-chain Y. One can imagine each of the two arms of the antibody molecule as made of double lines, like two equals (=) signs, tipped at 45-degree angles to each other. One line from each of the arms (the rest of the two heavy chains) extends downward to make the double-line trunk of the antibody.

By 1965 the complete amino acid sequence of the light chains from two different types of antibodies had been worked out. Part of the light chains from both molecules was identical, and the rest differed. This distinction led to the concept of light chains being made of two regions, variable (V) and constant (C). The same basic composition applies to the heavy chains, as well. The tips of the Y arms of the heavy chains are the variable regions. The rest of the two heavy chains, down to the "pillar" of the Y, is the constant region. The variable regions of the light and heavy chains lie next to each other, at the very tips of the arms of the Y.

Since the variable and constant regions of the light (and heavy) chains were seamlessly connected to one another in the molecule itself, it made sense to assume that one gene coded for the entire light chain. However, it was work by Lee Hood and others in the early 1960s that showed this was not the case. The *constant* regions of light chains were definitely the product of one gene. The variable regions, though, at least in mice, seemed to be the product of many different genes. This was what stimulated Bill Dreyer to propose the "two gene one polypeptide" theory.

In the late 1970s and early '80s, Susumu Tonegawa was focusing his research team's efforts on the genetic origin of light chains. In the series of brilliant experiments that eventually won him the Nobel Prize, he indirectly demonstrated that light chains have three rearranging elements: constant (C), for the constant region, and variable (V) and joining (J) elements for the variable region. These elements join together to create an antibody light chain. Meanwhile, Hood and his researchers were focused on the heavy chains. In many ways, he said to me, he felt they were more interesting. "We were the first to demonstrate that the variable regions of heavy chains had three separate regions that had to join together," said Hood. "Besides the V and J regions, there's a 'diverse' or D region. With the C region, that adds up to at least four regions for the heavy chain."

Hood and his lab team discovered the method by which three different genes, located in different places within a particular chromosome, combine to present the complete information needed to create the variable region of an antibody heavy chain. Imagine that the heavy chain is a copy of *War and Peace* existing in about 170 separate, hardbound parts, each part hidden somewhere on the shelves in the literature section of the Library of Congress. Finding those 170 segments, and then splicing them together in just the right order, is not an easy task. There are many different combinations that can be made—about ten thousand, in fact. Hood and his associates discovered how the human body performs this feat. The process of combining the different gene segments is called rearrangement, and it is irreversible. The B cell rearranges certain gene segments to make a heavy chain variable region for an antibody molecule. When it is finished, it's stuck with that specific arrangement. While an animal (human or otherwise) is still a fetus, millions of such rearrangements take place and create a pool of mature B cells. Each B cell is unique, committed to making a single unique antibody molecule.

Humans have about 150 variable gene segments, twelve

diverse segments, and six joining segments. That's about 10,000 different possible combinations—"combinatorial joinings," Hood called them—of V, D, and J segments encoding antibody heavy chain variable regions. Light chain variable regions are made of combinations of 150 V and six J segments, for about a thousand light chain sequences. The genetic card shuffling has begun. *Voila!* The beginning of antibody diversity.

And that *is* just the beginning, as Lee Hood pointed out to me. The immune system has several other kinds of shuffles it can do.

"Here are the fundamental mechanisms, up to now," said Hood. "You begin with a multiplicity of these gene elements. Then, you could generate diversity by putting about 150 V gene elements together with twelve D gene elements together with six or so J gene elements in all their different combinations. Once you have done this and expressed *them* as polypeptide chains, it turns out that you have a combinatorial level of amplification. This occurs because *any light chain can go together with any heavy chain*. So if you can make a thousand lights and ten thousand heavies, you've got the possibility of *ten million different antibody molecules*. That's two levels of combinatorial joining, of combinatorial diversity. OK?

"Next is a second kind of rearrangement for heavy chains, called *class switching*. This permits a particular D gene to be joined to any of the V genes by a second and very different kind of rearrangement. We demonstrated the existence of class switching." With this mechanism, a B cell cued early in its development to make one kind of antibody can shuffle D and V gene segments to "switch classes" and thus be able to make one of the other four major kinds of antibodies.

But there's still more, continued Hood; there are also

somatic mutational mechanisms. I started feeling over-
whelmed. Hood pressed on, undeterred. "There are two
kinds of these somatic-type mutations. First, the joining of
these gene segments—V, J, and D—can be imprecise. So
more diversity can be generated at the imprecisely joined
junctions. Secondly, there's a mechanism that David Baltimore demonstrated. You can actually throw in random
nucleotides, and then you join *these* things together. So
you have information that doesn't come from the organism's germ-line cells that's participating in the construction
of the gene."

Hood and his team were later among the first to
demonstrate convincingly the existence of still another
process called *hypermutation*. This takes place at a later
stage in the development of B cells. A somatic mutation
mechanism sprinkles the rearranged V gene mutations
through the genetic region coding for antibodies. One of
the examples Hood studied showed that 3 percent of the
nucleotides felt the action of this hypermutation process.
That didn't seem like much to me, but Hood demurred.
"Oh, no," he exclaimed. "That is very extensive, indeed."

In summary, several different mechanisms operate to
produce hundreds of millions of unique antibodies:

- The 170 or so different V, D, and J gene segments can
  be shuffled into more than 10,000 possible combinations, each a unique heavy chain variable region for an
  antibody.
- About 156 different J and V gene segments can
  combine into approximately 1,000 different light
  chain variable regions for an antibody.
- These 11,000 different light and heavy variable chains
  can combine together to create ten million different
  possible antibodies.

- Imprecise joining of the gene segments, which is one form of somatic mutation, produces still more possible unique antibodies.
- Another kind of somatic mutation, in which random nucleotides participate in the gene segment shuffles, causes still more unique antibodies to be created.
- Class switching, which takes place after the gene segments have been shuffled about and spliced together, allows the immune system to essentially change an antibody from one general type (there are five) to another.
- Finally, the hypermutation mechanism creates even more possibilities for the creation of new and unique antibody molecules.

Here, in sketchy form, is how these genetic shuffles occur and lead to the creation of antibody diversity—the hundreds of millions of possible antibodies which the body can call upon for help. Let's stick to the heavy chain variable region, studied and deciphered by Lee Hood and his research teams. The rearrangement of the heavy chain variable genes takes place during the development of B cells in the fetus. In humans, the genes for the heavy chains are located on chromosome 14. Random D and J genes (in that order) from different points on the DNA strand first join together during the process of genetic rearrangement in the fetal B cell. (The pieces of DNA that eventually are transcribed to messenger RNA are called *exons*. The intervening sequences of DNA, which are cut out and discarded, are called *introns*.) One segment of a variable heavy chain gene is joined to the D and J genes. The intervening introns get cut out of the DNA. The three randomly picked genes snuggle in together. Messenger RNA then transcribes the genetic information and carries it to a ribosome in the B cell. There is still genetic material between the J gene and the beginning of the gene for the heavy chain's constant region. It now gets cut away and discarded, so that the three genes for the variable region sit cheek-by-jowl with the gene for the constant region. The ribosome then begins translating into protein the completed gene for the heavy chain.

Hood leaned back in the leather-upholstered sofa and paused. "That must have been an exciting time," I remarked, speaking of the late 1970s and early 1980s, when his laboratory was breaking open the secret of antibody diversity. He nodded, remembering. "They *were* exciting times," he said, "So many things happened in such a short period of time. But the striking impression I have is how initially *misled* we were by an interesting observation whose meaning should have been apparent."

I shook my head. "Misled?"

"Yes," he replied. "Bill Dreyer's original hypothesis of 'two genes, one polypeptide chain' had the entire variable gene going down and joining up with the entire constant gene. When Tonegawa sequenced the first light chain gene, it was clear that it truncated somewhat early. There was a piece of the V region that was still missing. Yet nobody put it together that this was a *second* element, and *that* really was the locus of the joining, the rearranging. No one figured that out until, gosh, a year or year and a half later. It was an idea that is now so blatantly obvious, but that time we weren't programmed to think about it that way.

"Or for heavy chains, which we were working on, the concept that there was yet a *third* element—that really came out of protein sequence data that we generated. And that made it impossible to explain in any other way. Going and proving it at the DNA level was then a relatively straightforward thing to do. Actually, the element was the J and the D genes, so there were really two."

Still another puzzle stared Hood and his people in the

face for six months before they figured it out. Two different messenger RNAs seemed to exist for carrying the DNA coding for heavy chains over to the ribosomes. That didn't make sense. Why two messenger RNAs, when one would do nicely? They puzzled over it and poked at it. Finally, the answer became clear. It had to do with the fact that there are two different forms of antibodies. Some antibodies are secreted into the body, and float about in the body's fluids. Other antibodies remain bound to the membrane of the B cell, and act as receptors or molecular "locks" on the B cell's surface. In retrospect, said Hood, the answer was obvious once they thought about it. But it took a long time to recognize the obvious. The mechanism of RNA splicing was a brand new thing. It had just barely been described. This was the first example in the genes of higher organisms, where RNA splicing led to two forms.

Continued Hood: "Another thing that was really astounding when we discovered it, was the level that somatic hypermutation could operate at. Three percent of the nucleotides! That's a *staggering* amount. In fact, in most cases if you do take it that far, you probably destroy the gene's effectiveness. You change too much. It was just kind of"—Hood paused, at a loss for words—". . . the *wonderment* . . . of how. . . ." He shook his head. "We knew in a general sense the kind of things to expect. But the details were so much more clever and so much more sophisticated than we had ever appreciated initially. Nature had really done it much more nicely than we ever predicted."

"Was there ever a time," I asked, "when you'd be looking at some of this data—like, say, with hypermutation—and you just couldn't believe it? I mean, it was looking you in the face and it was obviously correct, but you just couldn't quite accept it?"

Hood grinned. "Oh, on the hypermutation thing we sequenced everything twice."

"You couldn't believe it."

"Yeah! We felt *very* uncomfortable with that.

"But, you know, *all* these things were difficult to accept. They stared us in the face for a long time. It's this whole business of a revolution of ideas in scientific thinking. You get fixed in simplistic models, and it takes a lot to break away. Each of these things was a wonderful new insight.

"And with each came this wonderment, of how incredibly elegant Nature had chosen to be."

I leaned back in my chair. "Was there any point at which referees of papers or editors of scientific journals just could not believe that this was really real?"

"Well, in the somatic hypermutation paper, for the first and only time in my life, we had to send in most of the sequencing gels. So the referee could read them." Hood laughed at the memory. "Really, can you believe it? He had to see the actual physical evidence to be convinced that there *were* that many mutations.

"But on the other hand, in a lot of cases—like RNA splicing, the third gene element—the data were so simple and the explanations so elegant, that as soon as they read it they said, 'Why, of *course!*'

"It was just getting to the point that you could *write* it that took a long time. You sit and sit and stare at it for a long time, and it *forces* itself upon you, the data *tears* you out of conventional patterns."

An analogy occurred to me, and I passed it on. "It's like being a flatland creature that has lived only in two dimensions, finally saying, well, by God there must be a third dimension."

Hood eyes lighted up. "*Exactly!* Exactly. And that is the ultimate dimension of pleasure in science. Realizing for the first time, *you know something that no one has ever understood before.*" He grinned hugely.

"I remember—and Phil Early really gets primary credit

for this—I remember when we first discovered there were these things called recognition sequences, that help to control all of the DNA rearrangements. These sequences of nucleotides are basically attached to the edges of the gene segments that rearrange. It's actually one or two turns of the DNA helix. There's enough diversity in these things that, again, it took a real genius of insight on the part of Phil Early to recognize these sequences, and then to understand what they meant. Ninety-nine out of a hundred scientists could look at that data and never have picked out those key fundamental patterns. Elegant experiments have since been done to prove these elements are the key elements in the whole rearrangement process.

"What most people don't realize, you see, is that DNA sequence data is enormously repetitive and monotonous. You've got your four basic subunits, and they repeat again and again and again. Being able to extract that information was just wonderful."

One misconception popularly held is that scientists like Lee Hood, who run university departments and head up laboratory research teams, actually do a lot of the "bench work" in an experiment. The truth is usually otherwise, Hood pointed out. "My interaction was all intellectual," he said. "By that time I had a lab of about fifteen or twenty people. It's my belief that once you get beyond five or six people, the amount of time you spend in the lab is minimal. Or you don't pay attention to the other things you have to do. The hands-on work was done by graduate students and postdocs.

"But that brings up something else," he continued. "One theme in all this work that has impressed me is that these major contributions were done by graduate students, doing this as their thesis work. And it was marvelous to see how unbounded and minimally constrained they were in analyzing and thinking about the data. They had relatively few preconceptions. As we get older we think we know more and more about how the world is, and it takes more and more to dissuade us of those convictions. Fresh young graduate students—their ignorance is what gives them their creativity."

Another theme that had jumped out at me during my time with Hood was that of elegance and simplicity. It appears in nearly every field of science, though it is particularly apparent in mathematics, cosmology, and physics. The *elegance* of a solution, its beauty or esthetic simplicity, is often what convinces a scientist that it is the *correct* solution.

Hood agreed. He found it particularly satisfying that a relatively small number of gene segments could produce an enormous number of unique antibodies. It was an elegantly simple solution to a serious problem confronting the immune system: How can it recognize and counteract an antigen that it has never seen before? That may have never even existed before? The answer is to scatter about the hundred or so gene segments that make this essential part of the immune system, instead of keeping them next to each other in the chromosomes. The different mechanisms of genetic shuffling are the essence of antibody diversity.

Lee Hood leaned forward over the table, with its books, journals, and metal sculpture. "It's a staggering concept to think of, isn't it," he said. "That nature could fashion these kinds of strategies to be able to interact with any kind of foreign antigen you might ever run into in the world. Just staggering."

2 The T Cell Army

John Farrar has about himself a sense of compressed energy. Even when he is obviously relaxed, leaning back in a chair in his office at Hoffmann-La Roche Inc.'s huge complex in Nutley, New Jersey—even then he exudes enthusiasm, his energy is barely contained. It struck me as the energy of excitement, of fun, perhaps even of born-again conversion. Farrar is a research immunologist turned corporate scientist. And he's quite obviously enjoying his second career as director of the department of immuno-pharmacology for a giant pharmaceutical company.

Farrar's career journey in some ways mirrors the journey that immunology is taking, from pure science to applied technology, from university and government laboratories to the labs of for-profit corporations. For John Farrar, for other immunologists and biologists turned entrepeneurs, and for the biotechnology industry at large, that journey has often traveled a road paved with T cells and their biochemical by-products.

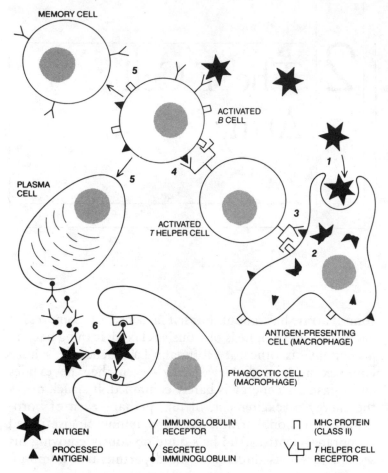

MEMORY CELL

ACTIVATED *B* CELL

PLASMA CELL

ACTIVATED *T* HELPER CELL

ANTIGEN-PRESENTING CELL (MACROPHAGE)

PHAGOCYTIC CELL (MACROPHAGE)

★ ANTIGEN	Y IMMUNOGLOBULIN RECEPTOR	⊓ MHC PROTEIN (CLASS II)
▲ PROCESSED ANTIGEN	Y● SECRETED IMMUNOGLOBULIN	*T* HELPER CELL RECEPTOR

The immune system's response to infection mobilizes many different cells. A macrophage (1) consumes the foreign antigen, then (2) digests the antigen and displays pieces of it on its surface. There a helper T cell recognizes it (3). The helper T cell does this by using receptors that recognize foreign antigens and Class II MHC proteins together. The now activated helper T cell activates B cells carrying the same antigen fragments (4). The B cells have antibody receptors on their surface, which detect the antigens. Some activated B cells become memory B cells (5), which will provide a swift response to future invasions. Others become plasma cells, which secrete antibodies that "tag" the antigen for destruction (6) by macrophages. *(From "The Molecules of the Immune System," © 1985 by Scientific American Inc. All rights reserved.)*

Since the early 1970s immunologists have realized that the immune system's ability to attack and destroy invading viruses depends on the class of immune system cells called T lymphocytes, or T cells. These cells also play an important role in the immune system's ability to deal with bacterial infections, but their most vital role is taking care of viruses and cells of the body that have been infected by viruses. The essential trigger for the T cell's antiviral ability is a molecule embedded in its surface. It goes by several names: "Cell-surface antigen" is one (for it can be, under certain circumstances, an antigen that triggers the immune system); "surface marker" (for they have been used to distinguish among different types of T cells) is another. In terms of its actual function, it may best be called a T cell *receptor*. For these molecules (and there are several) are essentially biochemical locks, and antigens from a virus are the keys that open the locks and unleash the destructive power of the T cell.

The B lymphocytes or B cells produce two kinds of complex protein molecules: antibodies and B cell receptors. The two are virtually identical in structure and composition. The main difference is that B cell receptors stay rooted in the B cell's surface membrane, and antibodies move around and through the blood and lymph. The immune system's antibodies are the active agents of the humoral immune response. They're ideally suited for dealing with infectious agents that float freely in the body's fluids.

T cells, on the other hand, seem to be designed to combat infections that are associated with the body's own cells. It's the T cells, the active agents of the cellular immune response, that attack and kill bodily cells that are cancerous or that have been infected and taken over by the various viruses. In order for antibodies to do their job, they need only be able to identify a cell or substance as

Not-Self. For the T cell, though, the task is more complicated. T cells must not only recognize a specific antigen as being an invader; they must also recognize that the antigen is associated with the infected Self host cell. The T cell must recognize *both* Self *and* Not-Self together. What's more, this kind of recognition has to stay under tight control. If T cells should be activated solely by Self molecules or proteins (which immunologists would call *autoantigens,* for "Self-antigens"), they would quickly turn against the body's own healthy cells and tissues. In fact, that is essentially what happens in the case of those diseases that are called *autoimmune* diseases—illnesses like multiple sclerosis, myasthenia gravis, and certain forms of diabetes and rheumatoid arthritis. In a real sense, the immune system is overreacting, attacking and killing cells that it should ignore.

John Farrar, like every other immunologist today, travels on a road built by others. The road to understanding the role of T cells, and how they function, is about fifty years long. It's been known for many decades that if tissue from one animal is grafted or transplanted to the body of a second animal, that second animal's immune system will reject the graft. The reason is straightforward: The second animal's immune system identifies the graft tissue as Not-Self and attacks it. But what is it about the foreign tissue that marks it as foreign? In the early 1930s an immunologist named Peter Gorer showed that tissue rejection was caused by the presence of molecules on the surface of the foreign tissue that were antigenic. Each person has a unique "Self-marker" on all of his or her cells. It's almost impossible that any two unrelated people will have identical Self-marker proteins. This is why organ transplants between two unrelated people with functioning immune systems always fail. Even children of the same parents have unique Self-markers on their cells. Only transplants between identical twins, whose Self-marker proteins are identical, stand an excellent chance of succeeding. Today that seems pretty obvious, but in the 1930s it was a major step forward in immunology.

Over the next twenty years, immunologists discovered that these Self-marker proteins are encoded by a special set of genes. These genes all lie close together in a DNA region called the *major histocompatibility complex,* or MHC. The prefix *histo-* means "tissue." In human beings the MHC is located in what's called the *human leukocyte antigen* (or HLA) complex. The HLA complex lies on the short arm of chromosome 6. The marker proteins made by the genes of the HLA complex are called *MHC-encoded proteins.* The MHC genes are remarkable in a number of ways, but one of the most amazing is their incredible diversity. There are literally millions of variants (or *alleles,* as geneticists would say) of the MHC genes. That in turn means there are millions upon millions of different MHC-encoded protein markers. And that's the reason why the odds against two unrelated people having identical MHC-encoded Self-marker proteins are literally astronomical.

In the 1950s the brilliant British scientist Sir Peter Medawar showed that the immune system's lymphocyte cells are the ones responsible for recognizing the Self-marker proteins on the surfaces of cells. He later went on to demonstrate ways of "fooling" the immune system into accepting transplants of foreign tissues. In 1960 Medawar received the Nobel Prize in Physiology or Medicine for his work. He shared the prize with the Australian doctor Sir Macfarlane Burnet, who had done similar work. Burnet later helped develop the clonal selection theory, which explained how a B cell makes millions of identical copies of itself and of an antibody against a specific antigen.

Still and all, there was considerable uncertainty about

the exact functions of MHC-encoded proteins. The uncertainty began to clear away in the 1960s with the work of people like Baruj Benacerraf of the U.S. National Institute of Allergy and Infectious Diseases, Hugh McDevitt of England's National Institute for Medical Research, and Michael Sela of the Weizmann Institute in Israel. Experiments by these three researchers revealed that the MHC genes affect the functions of T cells and not other immune system cells. It wasn't long before other immunologists suggested that the MHC genes actually carried the code for the T cell receptors. Subsequent experiments showed that MHC-encoded proteins also have some kind of interaction with foreign antigens, and that this interaction is a prerequisite for the actual functioning of the T cell receptor.

It turns out that a T cell pays attention to more than just an antigen. That antigen might be, say, from a virus, and it is being displayed on the surface of a host cell that's infected by that virus. The T cell receptor must also recognize and interact with some of the MHC-encoded Self-marking protein on the surface of that host cell. Only if it does both will the T cell go into action and begin the process that destroys the virus-infected cell. This phenomenon is called *MHC restriction*. The requirement that the T cell recognize the presence of both MHC-encoded proteins *and* an antigenic protein is what restricts the T cell's activity.

But for all the complexity of the MHC restriction phenomenon, it is only the beginning of the T cell's work. They do not operate in isolation, but in intricate cooperation with the rest of the immune system. John Farrar began his career in immunology, and his initial interest lay in the signals, the mechanisms, by which one subset of T cells regulated the response of the others.

Farrar's office could have been almost any of the ones I visited during my travels through the landscape of immunological research. Most were like his: small, crowded with shelves that were crowded with books and medical journals; a desk with piles of articles and magazines scattered across it; a couple of comfortable chairs, a table with more papers, and room to place a tape recorder and a plastic coffee cup. The coffee was mediocre, but hot. What made this office different from all the others was, of course, John Farrar. His presence dominated it.

As our conversation began, it was clear to me that Farrar was feeling a bit cautious. I imagined he was thinking: Who *is* this guy, anyway? What does he want to know? But he soon warmed to the subject, which at this point was the progress of his own career. Farrar was pleased with his professional journey, and he had every right to be. He had gone to work at the National Institutes of Health in 1972, and spent ten years doing fundamental research in lymphokine-guided regulation of the immune system. *Lymphokines* are the proteins that play a vital role in the immune system. The brain has neurotransmitter chemicals; the body's endocrine system has hormones; the immune system has lymphokines. Lymphokines are the chemical messengers of the immune system. They are the runners, the radio operators, who pass information from one group of soldiers to another. Ask anyone who has been in combat about how important the radio man is to a platoon. And as sometimes happens with a radioman in combat, some lymphokines can also kill the enemy.

"I started off in immunology," said Farrar, "with an interest in the signals, the mechanisms by which one group of T cells regulates the response of others. Even as a postdoc student, I was looking at how T cells turned on other cells." It was while working at the National Institutes of Health (NIH) that Farrar did research with a lymphokine that has since become famous. It's called *interleukin-2*, or IL-2. Interleukin-2 was initially called "human T cell growth factor" (TCGF). First discovered in 1968, it was purified and characterized in 1981 and 1982 by James W. Mier and Robert C. Gallo—the same Robert Gallo who would later codiscover the AIDS virus. Their work was done at NIH. "We demonstrated that IL-2 was involved in regulation of B and T cell responses," Farrar recalled. "My lab was one of the first, if not the first, to demonstrate that. Then I got involved in other chemicals, things like B cell growth factors and differentiation factors." These are the chemicals that spur the B cell to grow and turn into a plasma cell and begin releasing its unique brand of antibodies.

Farrar spent ten years working on that very fundamental research. But by 1981 and 1982 it all started to seem endless. It was, he said, like working on a jigsaw puzzle. "I realized I could spend thirty more years of my life filling in other pieces of the puzzle, churning out paper after paper. The puzzle would get bigger and bigger, but I really couldn't see a practical application to what I was doing.

"I decided that it would be worthwhile to try doing something practical with this body of knowledge. And I realized that to really do something practical, you have to have the resources to do it. The things we are trying to do are really quite distinct from the things that a basic, fundamental immunologist will do." So John Farrar came to Hoffmann-La Roche.

Farrar's path began in basic research. For both B cells and T cells, the path to maturity begins in the bone marrow, with pluripotent stem cells. B cells branch out of them and eventually come to maturity in the body itself. The presence of the right antigen spurs a B cell to convert into a plasma cell and begin making antibodies.

For T cells, however, the path is different. T lymphocytes undergo further development in the thymus gland, located underneath the breastbone. T-cell development in the thymus begins in the fetus and continues throughout a person's life. The T lymphocyte precursor cells migrate from the bone marrow to the thymus, and there they are processed in a way that is still not entirely understood. In the thymus the T cells develop on their surfaces the complex molecules called variously cell-surface antigens, surface markers, or T cell receptors, and finally become able to function in the immune system.

As the T cells develop in the thymus, different surface markers appear and disappear in their surfaces. By discovering the existence, development, and loss of these various markers, immunologists have begun tracing out the T cell's journey to maturity. At various stages of its development, T cells are called thymocytes and common thymocytes. Eventually they mature into one of at least three known major kinds of T cells:

• *Helper T cells* account for 55 to 70 percent of all the T cells. They do just what their name says: They help other immune system cells to multiply into a huge clone and swing into action against invaders. Helper T cells have a particular kind of molecule on their surfaces, a cell-surface marker called the CD4 receptor.

• *Cytotoxic or killer T cells* actually kill cells that have been infected by invading viruses. They latch onto the cell's surface and inject a chemical into it. The chemical causes the cell's surface to develop holes, and the cell dies.

• *Suppressor T cells* slow down and eventually stop the proliferation of other immune cells and immunological chemicals. They bring the immune reaction to a halt when the invading germs or viruses have been destroyed. Suppressor and killer T cells carry a marker on their surface called CD8. They account for 25 to 40 percent of all T cells.

Different kinds of T cells recognize the presence of different types of MHC-encoded proteins. In general, cytotoxic or killer T cells recognize a group called class I proteins. Class I proteins are present on the surfaces of every single cell in the human body—all 100 trillion of them. Helper T cells are also MHC-restricted. However, these T cells, with their CD4 receptors, recognize a different class of MHC-encoded proteins called class II proteins. In humans, class II proteins are found *only on T cells, B cells, macrophages,* and a few specific cells of other kinds of tissues. This is what makes it possible for helper T cells to "see" and activate these specific other immune cells.

And where does interleukin-2 fit into all this? IL-2 is a vital link in the immune response. IL-2 interacts with killer T cells by binding to specific membrane receptors. The receptors are *not* present on inactive mature T cells. They appear only after the T cell has been kicked into action. When IL-2 and its receptor on the killer T cells are both present, the killer T cells proliferate. Both must be present for this to happen. If either is missing, the killer Ts will cease growing and dividing, and will die. What's more, IL-2 receptors quickly disappear from the T cells' surfaces when the triggering antigen is gone. This is a simple yet effective "brake" on the continuing growth of killer T cells in response to invasion. The system *requires* the continuing stimulation by an antigen to react.

Unraveling the nature and structure of B cell receptors and immunoglobulins, while difficult, was made easy by the fact that activated B cells make huge amounts of identical antibodies. So do some kinds of cancerous tumors. Access to a lot of identical immunoglobulins made the task of deciphering and mapping the structure of antibodies a relatively easy task.

Figuring out the actual structure of T cell receptors was much more difficult. T cells, unlike B cells, do not produce antibodies or anything analogous to them. They simply carry their receptors on their surface, and there are not a lot of receptors, either. Many researchers at first assumed that there would be some way to get T cells to make a lot of antibodylike molecules. However, by the early 1970s it was pretty apparent that this wasn't going to happen. Another method would have to be found to figure out the structure of the T cell receptors.

Two major breakthroughs finally made the nearly impossible possible. The first took place in the early 1970s, and it was a truly revolutionary one. Cesar Milstein and Georges Kohler, working at the Medical Research Council's Laboratory of Molecular Biology in Cambridge, England, found a way to make immortal B cells that continually produced huge quantities of identical antibodies. They fused a B cell with a cancerous tumor cell to make something new: a B cell *hybridoma*. Cancer cells are by nature immortal: They continually grow and divide, grow and divide, consuming the body's food, energy, and resources. A B cell hybridoma has the immortality of the cancer cell, and the antibody-secreting ability of the activated B cell. It continually grows and make antibodies. The antibodies are all identical—thus the term *monoclonal antibodies*. Kohler and Milstein shared the 1984 Nobel Prize in Medicine or Physiology for their work. (Also sharing in that year's medical Nobel was Niels Jerne, who developed the idiotype theory of immune networks.)

The second breakthrough connected Kohler's and Milstein's advance with the T cell receptor problem. Over a period of several years in the mid-1970s, several teams of researchers developed ways to make T cell hybridomas for specific antigens and MHC-encoded Self-proteins. These hybridomas, what's more, could be grown in tissue cultures. This second breakthrough, coupled with the monoclonal antibody breakthrough, made it possible for research teams to make specific antibodies *targeted for specific T cell receptors.*

That breakthrough made two things possible. First, researchers could now begin telling apart the different kinds of T cells based on their different receptors. For example, this is what made it possible to say that the helper T cell is distinguished by the presence of the CD4 receptor. And that, in turn, led to a major finding about how people become infected with AIDS. Secondly, researchers could begin figuring out the actual chemical and physical structure of the T cell receptor. The tight chemical bond between the antibodies and the T cell receptor made it possible for researchers to purify relatively large quantities of T cell receptor for the first time. The quantities were finally large enough for them to begin deciphering its molecular and structural properties.

The picture of the T cell receptor's structure began to unfold from 1982 through 1985. Much of the significant work in this area was performed by researchers led by the husband-and-wife team of John Kappler and Phillipa Marrack at the National Jewish Center for Immunology and Respiratory Medicine in Denver, Colorado. Other important players included Mark Davis, who had moved from Lee Hood's lab to a position at Stanford University, Tak Mak, at the Ontario Cancer Institute, Haruo Saito and Susumu Tonegawa at the Massachusetts Institute of Technology, and Lee Hood.

Perhaps not too surprisingly, the T cell receptor resembles in some ways the antibody molecule. The T cell receptor also has a structural resemblance to both class I and class II MHC-encoded proteins. The T cell receptor, like the antibody molecule, is made of two polypeptide chains, which are coded for by separate genes. The chains, called the *alpha* and *beta* chains, are held together by sulphide bonds—also like the antibody chains. The receptor is always found in close association with the CD3 marker. All of these proteins—class I, class II, T cell receptor, and antibody—have loops made of about seventy amino acids embedded in each chain. Like antibody molecules, the two chains of the T cell receptor have constant (C), diversity (D), joining (J), and variable (V) regions. Each such region is encoded by distinct and separate segments of DNA in the genome.

John Farrar followed closely the developments leading to greater understanding of T cell receptors. He too was interested in certain receptors on the surfaces of T cells. He may have been in the middle of changing his career, but his interests had remained the same.

"And how," I asked him, "does a seasoned immunological researcher at NIH get together with a multinational drug company?"

"Well," Farrar said with a smile, "it was a case of a little bit of them looking for me and me looking for them. I was invited to a workshop that Roche had set up for immunologists, to tell them what was hot in immunology, where there are opportunities, and so on. That was in February 1982. Six months later there were a bunch of headhunters out looking for people.

"I came here in November of 1982. Hoffmann-La Roche had an interest in immunology. David Webb was at the Roche Institute [the research arm of Hoffmann-La Roche], and he was the only immunologist with the institute. He had done some work on suppressor lymphokines and on compounds called prostaglandins. But the company's main thrust with immunology was with immunodiagnostics. So the head people made a decision to move into immunopharmacology. They established a department of immunopharmacology. I applied and came on board as its director."

For Farrar, there was a curious side story to his employment by Hoffmann-La Roche. The company had set up a collaboration with the Immunex Corporation, a small genetic engineering company in Seattle, to get some supplies of interleukin-2. Farrar said, "I had interviewed with Immunex in 1981. They were telling me all their grand plans, and they were looking for a big company to work with. I had said that was interesting—and they *were* interesting—but it never worked out.

"So one year later I came to Hoffmann-La Roche—and ended up working with Immunex."

When Farrar first came to Roche, interleukin-2 was not the central theme of his new department. His years at NIH had been at the very beginnings of lymphokine therapy. Dudley Dumond and others were just starting to put lymphokines into people. They were crude mixtures, really, not purified at all. They were being given to cancer patients, and always with the idea of enhancing the immune response. When Farrar arrived in Nutley, New Jersey, at the end of 1982, bringing his lymphokine orientation with him from NIH, his initial thought was, "Well, La Roche has IL-2 started, so I'll bring along IL-3, IL-4, IL-5, and so on." In fact, it's now up to interleukin 7, and counting. (IL-7 was discovered in 1988 by the Immunex Corporation.) But Farrar did not head in that direction. A clinical immunologist named Paul Nadler changed his thinking.

"Nadler told me, 'Clearly there are opportunities for lymphokines to enhance the immune response. But the really major medical problems are not associated with immunodeficiency. In terms of the absolute numbers of people, they're associated with an *overactive* immune response.' And he went through a list of fifty to sixty diseases. And it really is that long.

"In terms of immunodeficiencies," he said, "you have, first and foremost, viral-induced immune deficiency— AIDS. You also have some naturally occuring, spontaneous genetic disorders, which are referred to as SCIDS—Severe Combined Immune Deficiency Syndrome." A Texas youngster known only as David the Bubble Boy was probably the most famous SCIDS patient. "And then there are what's called *iatrogenic*, or physician-induced, immune deficiencies. These for the most part are immune deficiencies that are an unavoidable side effect of chemotherapy and radiation therapy for cancer. That probably represents the biggest batch of immunodeficiencies.

"*But*," said Farrar with emphasis, "in terms of absolute numbers, immune deficiency diseases pale in comparison to the numbers of people with overactive systems."

Nadler convinced Farrar that the thrust of his new department at Roche should not be trying to boost immune responses, but rather to set up programs that could *slow down* overactive immune systems. The question, of course, was, How do you do that? It wasn't difficult to come up with some very sophisticated ways of doing this—which would take fifteen years to bring to a drug. But Farrar wasn't at NIH anymore. He was at Hoffmann-La Roche, Incorporated. His research had to produce a drug, and he would not have unlimited amounts of time in which to do it. He wouldn't have to drop his research on interleukin-2, but redirect his focus.

How, exactly, does interleukin-2 work? Basically, like this:

An invading antigen enters the body, and a macrophage finds it and eats it. The macrophage displays a piece of invading antigen on its surface. Some helper T cells and killer T cells come along. The marvelous mechanism of MHC restriction comes into play. Out of the hundreds of millions of T cells in the body, these particular helper and killer T cells recognize the macrophage as Self and its displayed foreign antigen as Not-Self. They both bind themselves to the macrophage and pieces of its displayed antigen. The macrophage now begins secreting interleukin-1, the first chemical messenger in the sequence. IL-1 triggers the mature helper T cell to change into an *effector* or activated helper T. The now-activated T cell begins to grow and divide, making identical copies—clones—of itself. It also starts releasing interleukin-2.

Meanwhile, the mature killer T cell has also bound to the macrophage and an exposed piece of antigen. That causes the killer T to grow IL-2 receptors on its surface. The interleukin-2 being released by the activated helper T cell and its identical clones in turn activates the killer T cell. It now begins to grow, divide, and produce clones of itself. The next generations of activated helper Ts, identical clones of the original T cell that "recognized" the antigen as foreign, also grow, divide, and release IL-2. The entire process begins to grow into a torrential immune response. The IL-2 continues to be pumped out, stimulating the succeeding generations of killer T cell clones. A "cascade effect" is taking place. This continues until the killer T cells have, through their own processes, destroyed the invading antigens. Once the infected cells are all gone, the IL-2 receptors begin to disappear from the surfaces of the T cells. The killer T cells stop growing and dividing, and die. Suppressor T cells slow down and stop the continuing production of helper T cells (which have also been urging the B cells to create antibodies). The immune response and its lymphokine cascade comes to a halt. The invaders have been defeated.

The discovery of IL-2, and the information discovered about how it works, would prove to be invaluable to the pharmaceutical industry. IL-2 and the other lymphokines would eventually be produced by genetic engineering and put to use in a myriad of new drugs and chemical compounds. But as Farrar began his work at Hoffmann-La Roche, those advances were still in the future. Farrar was thinking about shorter-term goals. "When I was at NIH," Farrar recalled as I flipped the cassette in my recorder, "I began to see this exodus of people from academia heading to the drug companies. And I heard stories about Howard Rosenthal, who had gone from NIH to Merck. I had known him at NIH. Well, the story was, Rosenthal was telling people: 'You get into industry, you got five years; you better have a drug in five years, or—pssht!—you're out!'

"So this is in the back of my head, right? And I can think of all these fancy, sophisticated schemes to come up with the perfect immunosuppressive drug. But I was being challenged to come up with some *short-term* programs. 'Give us something here and now, not the most sophisticated thing, but something that will be the bread and butter.' The question I was asking myself was, 'What can I put on the table soon, in order to support longer-term research programs?' Something I could take to the top and say, 'Here we are, this will make us some money—and look what I've got coming up next!' "

Farrar and his new department put together a program based simply on looking at some of Roche's own chemicals. The company had over the years compiled an enormous collection of organic compounds—a chemical library of immense size and complexity. It is the Library of Congress of organic chemical collections. Many of them had never been tested in any thorough manner. They had simply been discovered (or created in a laboratory) and then scientifically described. A small amount of the compound was then stored in some vault or room somewhere. Farrar's approach was simple and straightforward. "We simply began testing organic compounds in Roche's collection, compounds whose chemical description sounded promising." He grinned. "And damned if it didn't work out! We found some very potent organic compounds with powerful immunosuppressive properties, in vitro and in vivo. In fact now we have one. It has been recommended for clinical development, and it is more potent than Cyclosporin A."

Cyclosporin A is an immunosuppressive drug derived from a mushroom. It has gotten a lot of coverage in the popular press, because it is used for organ transplantation. Cyclosporin A virtually shuts down the immune system, so that the body can safely accept a new heart, liver, or kidney from some other body. Cyclosporin A is very powerful, and is pretty much the drug of choice for organ transplant patients.

Disrupting the release of IL-2 can lead to serious problems. Too much IL-2 can lead to an overactive immune response—the kind of problem that Paul Nadler was urging John Farrar to focus on. Too little IL-2, on the other hand, can cause immunosuppression. Cyclosporin A acts by preventing certain activated T cells from releasing IL-2. In other words, Cyclosporin A is an interleukin-2 inhibitor.

However, as Farrar pointed out, Cyclosporin A is not without its problems. "It's state-of-the-art, all right," he said, "and it's not as great as it was originally cracked up to be. It's terribly toxic. When you are using therapeutic doses, you are using toxic doses. It does terrible things to your liver. And that is state of the art? That tells you where we are today. This stuff [his recent discovery] is better. It's more effective and less toxic. And it is very potent. We think we have a therapeutic index." (Determine the safe maximum tolerated dose, and also the safe minimum cumulative dose. Then divide the number for the former by the number for the latter. The result is the therapeutic index for the drug.) "We can use it in animals without toxic effects."

"What is it?" I asked.

"Well, I can't go into a lot of detail," said Farrar. "But—well, I can tell you that it's called 'RO-236457.' It's a derivative of vitamin A, or a retinoid compound."

"And how long did it take you to come up with it?"

"This we came up with in about three years. And it will probably go into humans, in clinical trials, in the fall of 1987. First in transplant patients, and then autoimmune diseases."

RO-236457 was Farrar's short-term project, the one that would hopefully put bread and butter on the table, and convince his superiors that he had the right stuff for the long haul. The project turned out to be a good one; by the summer of 1988 the clinical trials on RO-236457 were progressing well, and the drug showed great potential. For the long term, Farrar's department is looking for chemicals that act to block the action of interleukin-1, interleukin-2, and other lymphokines. This is the high-tech program, said Farrar. "It's liable to come up with new approaches or potential therapeutics that are more specific and less toxic. But it will take a much longer time to reach fruition."

Farrar's researchers are looking for ways to prevent IL-1, IL-2, and their chemical cousins from interacting with T cells and B cells. These cells have a "lock," a receptor molecule, into which the lymphokine "key" fits. Farrar wants to plug the locks. Interleukin-2 helps kick the immune response into high gear. By preventing it from doing its thing, Farrar would achieve his goal of slowing down overactive immune systems. It could lead to a major breakthrough in treating autoimmune diseases and other

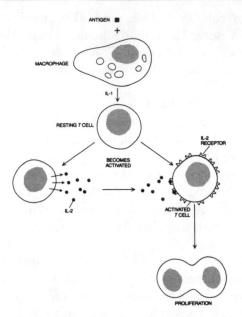

The response of T cells to infection depends on the release of proteins called interleukin 1 (IL-1) and interleukin 2 (IL-2). When a macrophage encounters and digests a foreign antigen it releases IL-1. The IL-1, in turn, causes T cells to release IL-2 and to grow IL-2 receptors on their surfaces. The IL-2 "key" fits the receptor "lock," stimulating the T cells to grow, divide, and mature into fully functioning T cells. *(From "The First Human Retrovirus," © 1986 by Scientific American American Inc. All rights reserved.)*

illnesses caused by an overactive immune response. To get there, though, Farrar and his people have first to accomplish two specific tasks. First, they would have to use genetic engineering techniques to clone the genes that code for each lymphokine receptor. They would also have to clone the genes that carry the instructions to make IL-1 and IL-2. Second, they would have to get these genes to make actual proteins. Once those two tasks were done, said Farrar, they would look for the IL-1 and IL-2 inhibitors in two different ways.

"First," he said, "you can take a very empirical approach. A shotgun approach, if you will. You look at the interaction of the proteins, and then start screening everything and its brother to see if they inhibit the binding. Or you can use a more rational approach. You determine the actual three-dimensional structure of *this* protein and then *this* one. You figure out how they interact, what amino acid residues are touching each other and interacting. You get the three-dimensional structure of the groove where they interact. Then you design a drug that fits into that groove and blocks it."

"Which approach are you taking?"

Farrar smiled at me. "Oh, we're taking both ways—the shotgun approach and the rational design approach," Farrar replied. "There are proponents of both methods and opponents of both methods. But it's a healthy competition. And I find it interesting to watch, and to guide it and keep it under control."

I had to laugh, in admiration of the strategy. It was cunning, I thought. It was also expensive. Hoffmann-La Roche didn't have unlimited amounts of money, but the company certainly had more resources than did an academic researcher, or perhaps even someone working at a government-run laboratory. The simultaneous two-track approach Farrar's group was running would not be an option for a lot of researchers in academia or the government.

"Give me an example of how this kind of long-range program might work at Hoffmann-La Roche," I asked him. So he did. It had to do with obesity. An enzyme made by the pancreas breaks down lipids—fatty substances—in the intestines, so they can be absorbed by the body. If that enzyme could be inhibited, then lipids would not be broken down and wouldn't be absorbed by the body. Such an enzyme inhibitor would be a possible antiobesity compound. One project at Roche involved the tedious long-term screening of different compounds for inhibitors of this enzyme. In the end, the company came up with a promising compound that eventually went into clinical trials as an antiobesity drug.

Farrar's search of interleukin antagonists was taking him back to Roche's drug library, but also further than that. "Yes, we are looking at organic compounds from Roche's file, and also at compounds from other companies on contract. We're looking at natural compounds, extractions of oak leaves, for example. You know, a chemist would never dream up some of the types of structures that come out of natural sources."

The rational approach was progressing quite nicely. "Interleukin-2 comes in two different chemical versions," he said, "and we already had both of the relevant proteins. We have now cloned the IL-2 gene and have expressed the IL-2 receptor. That's the first time that's been done all the way through. Now we're in the process of identifying the chemical residues. That's part of the task of identifying the three-dimensional structure of the receptor." Knowing the receptor's three-dimensional structure would be like knowing what the inside of a lock looks like. If you know that, you can figure out how the key works—and how to *block* the key from working.

It struck me that the shotgun approach, though possibly fruitful in the long run, would be very tedious and time-consuming. "Well, the random approach is actually being done by robots," said Farrar. "A computer-driven robot runs these assays. We have one technician that sits there and pushes a button, and the robot's arm swings around above these assays and does them. Now, that's the type of thing which could probably only be done by a pharmaceutical company."

The random approach, too, was already having some results. Farrar's people had found some compounds that inhibit IL-2. The questions still to be answered were, Are they powerful enough? And will they inhibit IL-2 in a biological system—a living creature instead of a test tube? To answer those questions would take time. A lot of time. How much more time? I asked. "Oh, maybe five years," Farrar replied. "Five to seven years. I called this a seven-to-ten-year project when we started, and we started in 1984. So five to seven more years."

He gave me some more detail on the time line. "I think from the time from when you identify something in the random search, it takes about six months to a year to isolate the actual compound. Nine times out of ten all that will give you is a structural lead. Chemists will then work for two years to synthesize the compound and also some analogs, compounds with similar structures, with simultaneous evaluation of them in vitro and also in living biological systems.

"Then you'll spend maybe two more years doing the end-stage evaluation to get it ready to recommend for clinical trials, which can take another year. So, really, you're literally talking five to seven years."

Farrar paused for a moment and looked through some papers on his desk and found what he was looking for. He said, "Recently we had a management conference here, and my group did a theoretical exercise. We took a drug from discovery through to commercialization. We began with the premise that it was first discovered in-house, over at the Roche Institute. Then we took it all the way through. You know how long it added up to?

"*Fourteen years*. And we also figured out how many people would be involved—128 man-years over a fourteen-year period of time.

"That's what we're doing."

3 Communications and Cancer

On August 12, 1986, my friend Juliana Moon died. She was in her late sixties. The cause of death was cancer. I forget now where it began—the breast, I think, before I met her. At first it seemed that surgery and radiation stopped it. But no such luck. Tumor cells had migrated to her spine. Then other bones. Then the brain. She hung on and hung on, a woman of laughter, a woman of compassion, a woman of strength. My wife, who met her only once, later spoke of her with awe in her voice as "a wise woman." The tumor neither knew nor cared. It merely grew. And finally killed.

Three months later another friend of mine died of cancer. Peggie Wolfson was only in her midforties, mother of three children, the youngest still in high school. In Peggie's case it was lung cancer, which spread to her liver. She also suffered from lupus, an autoimmune disease that had left her immune system functioning below par in the first place. That limited the kinds of treatments that could be used for the tumor. The time from diagnosis to her death was less than a year. I was thirty-seven at the time. They were the first friends of my adult life to die.

Three thousand miles away, researchers at a company in Cambridge, Massachusetts, were working on new techniques to fight and defeat the kinds of cancers that killed my friends. Genetics Institute, Inc. (GI), is a new breed of corporation—a biotechnology company. These upstarts in the medical-pharmaceutical business are using state-of-the-art genetic engineering technology to create new medical therapies for a myriad of diseases. Arthritis, multiple sclerosis, cancers, genetic disorders, AIDS—all are targets of biotech companies.

My introduction to GI came from Robert Kamen, the company's director of research. The company's story had begun eight years earlier. In 1978 Derek Bok, the president of Harvard University, thought it would be a good idea for the university to start up a biotech company. The university spent a lot of time looking at it, and Bok finally asked Mark Ptashne to check it out. Ptashne is one of the most brilliant of the new breed of biologists who have created the field of genetic engineering. Ptashne got very excited about the idea and put together a proposal. Bok in turn took it the Harvard faculty and put it up to a vote—and they turned it down.

"That was a very good decision by them," Kamen told me one winter afternoon. "I think it would have been totally inappropriate for Harvard to be running a company." I had come to Kamen's office near Cambridge to talk about immune system chemicals and how they are being put to commercial medical use. He was eager to talk about the various products GI has in the commercial pipeline, but first he gave some background on the company. It was an interesting story. Genetics Institute might never have come into existence if the Harvard faculty had accepted Ptashne's and Bok's plan for an in-house biotech company.

Ptashne, Kamen recalled, was in a bind. Harvard had left him in the lurch, and he didn't know the first thing about starting a company. A friend of Ptashne, a business consultant, then introduced him to one of her friends, a man who had once started his own company that had done quite well. The man was William Paley, and the company he started was CBS.

"Well, Paley loved the idea of a biotech company," said Kamen. "Ptashne said he'd start up the company if Paley would be on the board of directors. Paley told him that was just fine. Ptashne then said, 'Great. Let's get rid of all these venture capitalists, and you help me raise some money.' And Paley said, 'No, no, those guys are all close friends of mine.' "

Within a week Ptashne had a check for $6 million. Genetics Institute, Inc., was born. Ten years later it was booming, and the products in its development pipeline included genetically engineered immune system chemicals for fighting cancer.

"Cancer" is the common name for a malignant neoplasm or tumor. *Neoplasm* literally means "new growth." There are two kinds of neoplasms, benign and malignant tumors. A malignant tumor invades surrounding structures and spreads (or *metastasizes*) to distant parts of the body. A benign tumor stays put. *Sarcomas* are cancers that occur in bone, muscle, and connective tissues—the so-called mesenchymal tissues. *Carcinomas* are cancers that originate in the skin, mucous membrane cells, or glandular tissues. Sarcomas metastasize through the bloodstream. Carcinomas usually spread through the lymphatic system.

The precise causes of most kinds of cancers are unknown. What *is* known, though, is that there are clear connections between environmental factors and some cancers. The most obvious is the link between cigarette smoking and lung cancer. Exposure to asbestos is clearly connected to some kinds of cancers of the cells lining the lung cavities. A combination of cigarette smoking and alcohol consumption is causally linked to stomach cancer, cancer of the esophagus, and oral cancer. Uranium and nickel miners have a much higher than normal incidence of lung cancer. Exposure to some plastic compounds is related to development of tumors in blood vessels.

However, not all cancers have an exclusively environmental cause or connection. Researchers in recent years have clearly established the existence of a genetic component to cancers. That is, some people seem to be genetically predisposed to contracting some cancers. And some cancers may actually have genetic rather than environmental causes.

Finally, evidence now exists for viruses as the cause of some cancers. Scientists have known for years that some malignancies in animals were caused by viruses. It is now known that some human cancers are also virus-caused. Robert Gallo of the National Cancer Institute, who later found worldwide fame (and controversy) for his codiscovery of the AIDS virus, discovered the first virus known to cause a human cancer. It's named HTLV-I, for Human T-Lymphotrophic Virus One. It causes cancer of T cells.

The traditional pharmaceutical corporations have always been quick to take the basic research findings of people like Gallo and turn them into usable drugs and medical treatments. They've got the money and the human resources to do it. The new generation of biotech companies are also making quick use of scientific discoveries made in academic and government labs. But the biotech industry is very different from many other new industries. Anyone familiar with the pharmaceutical industry knows it can take at least ten years before a biotech company will really show a profit. If those who had first started biotech companies really knew what they were getting into at the time, they probably would have stayed right were they were. Many of them were scientists, who didn't understand that there is a six-to-ten-year cycle to get a biological product from idea to the marketplace. Hoffmann-La Roche, for example, began work on its genetically engineered version of interferon (called Roferon) in 1979. It didn't come onto the market until 1986—a development time of seven years.

But despite the long lead times and frequent financial insecurity of being involved in the biotech industry, Bob Kamen was happy with his lot. "Not only is this work beneficial to people," he said, "but it's *fun*. This is very exciting work. What we're working on here at Genetics Institute is very interesting and difficult, and has tremendous social benefit. It's very different from working in certain other high-tech industries, where your major client is the government, and what you're working on, one way or another, is killing people. I wouldn't particularly enjoy that."

Kamen's journey to GI was in many ways similar to that of John Farrar at Hoffmann-La Roche. "I was working with the Imperial Cancer Research Fund in England," he recalled. "I was getting a little bored, I guess. I wrote a lot of research papers. I trained a lot of students. And I was ready for a change. There's a fellow named Tom Leonadis, who's a friend of mine and who was Mark Ptashne's grad student. I met Ptashne at a scientific meeting, and we ended up having lunch. He asked me if I'd be interested in getting involved in his new company, so I came to Boston and looked it over. That was in 1982. They had about forty people working for the company. Now there are over 300."

GI, Kamen explained, is a research organization that decided to become a fully integrated biotech company. The first thing the company did was to license a lot of their products to different companies. The reason was to solve the economic problem: How do you build a large R & D company without eating up a lot of your equity? It turned out to be a good move. GI built itself a very solid R & D base—one larger than nearly any other biotech company. Genentech, located in south San Francisco, is currently the world's largest biotech corporation. In distant second place is Amgen, headquartered in Thousand Oaks, California (where I coincidentally had attended college in the late 1960s). Genetics Institute is either Number Three or Number Four, depending on how one figures these things. Genentech is fifteen times larger than Amgen and the sixth largest pharmaceutical company in the world, with a valuation of over $4 billion.

"Four *billion* dollars? That's insane!" I said.

Kamen answered sharply, "No, actually that's not insane. It's very justifiable by very conservative financial analysis. Their valuation as a company is largely based on one product—their synthetic growth hormone, which looks good. They are also number one with another genetically engineered compound called *tPA*, which is *tissue plasminogen activator*. We're working on tPA, too, but Genentech will market it first, without any doubt." tPA is a compound that prevents blood clots from forming in a person's circulatory system. It has had dramatic effects in reducing second heart attacks in people who are still suffering the effects of a first heart attack.

Synthetic growth hormone, synthetic human insulin, and a few other compounds were in the first generation of genetically engineered medicines. Tissue plasminogen activator (tPA) is among the second generation of genetically engineered medicines. The next generation will include compounds that will revolutionize the treatment of cancers by improving the ability of the patient's immune system to attack and destroy the tumor. This is called *immunotherapy*. Molecules on the surface and in the interior of tumor cells can be recognized by the immune system as being different from what is normal. That is, the immune system identifies them as Not-Self and attacks them. These are called *tumor-associated antigens*. The cytotoxic or killer T cells attack tumor cells directly and destroy them. Other T cells bring in macrophages to do the deed. Natural killer cells, which are not antigen-specific like T cells and antibodies, also kill tumor cells. Antibodies help in fighting cancer cells by binding to them and bringing them into contact with killer Ts.

However, the malignant cells are also able to use the immune system to their own advantage. Chemical compounds released by the tumor cells stimulate the production of suppressor T cells. Normally the suppressor Ts go into action at the end of a battle against an invading antigen. They slow down and eventually stop the immune response when it is no longer needed. In this case, though, the tumor cells kick suppressor T cell production into high gear, shutting down (or at least slowing) the immune response early in the battle. The immune system is thus crippled, and unable to mount an effective attack against the tumor. As the tumor grows, so does its effectiveness in slowing down the immune response. The major aim of immunotherapy, therefore, is to boost (or supplement) the immune system's anticancer elements, without further stimulating the suppressor T cells.

But there's a significant problem with using some immune system compounds for cancer treatment: their toxicity. Cancer-killing doses are often poisonous to the patient. Nontoxic doses, though, aren't strong enough to kill substantial numbers of tumor cells. It can be a case of "damned if you do, and damned if you don't."

It was lunchtime, and I was ready for a boost to my digestive system. Lunch consisted of sliced turkey sandwiches with mayonnaise and lettuce on white bread, potato chips, a pickle, and a can of Pepsi Cola. It looked as if it had come from a vending machine. I didn't complain. I was hungry, and it was free.

Between bites, Kamen talked some more about then and now at GI. He had originally been approached by Ptashne and Leonadis to work as a researcher. At that point, he said, they hadn't thought they'd need someone to be director of research. But it became clear after about a year that they would in fact need someone to fill that niche. So they hired Kamen to organize the research arm of the company and provide a little bit of "mature leadership": He was five years older than the others. A typical day for Kamen (his official title is "senior vice president of scientific affairs") is now spent talking to people. Kamen spends a lot of time in meetings, dealing with scientific issues, business issues, inventory, and what he called "political stuff." He doesn't do research anymore. He's a communicator, essentially, and a facilitator of communications among researchers, management types, accountants, and —at times—science writers.

Communications, of course, is the real name of the game for the immune system. If the different parts of the immune system cannot "talk" to one another, the entire system collapses. A variety of naturally occurring substances perform this vital role. There may be dozens of these chemicals. They are among the most intensely studied compounds in immunology today. They're also very "hot" in biotechnology, because some of them are going to make some people very rich. And other people well again.

One set of chemicals, called *eicosanoids,* play a small but significant role in the immune system. Two kinds of eicosanoids are particularly interesting: *leukotrienes* and *prostaglandins.* There are several different kinds of each, and they have various roles in the body. Of interest to immunologists—and to anyone who's had a splinter in his finger, for that matter—is that these compounds are involved in the inflammatory response. That's the medical term for the redness and swelling that happens at the site of the splinter in your finger, or the cut on my hand. One leukotriene, called leukotriene B_4 or LTB_4, causes the immune system cells called neutrophils and eosinophils to congregate at the site of an infection. These cells are among the front-line troops of the immune system, the first into the breach against the infection.

Prostaglandins and leukotrienes don't get much attention in the popular press. But some other proteins, called *lymphokines,* have. Lymphokines are not antibodies, but rather are proteins secreted by lymphocytes that have been activated by the presence of an antigen. These chemicals perform for the immune system functions similar to those performed by hormones for the endocrine system, or neurotransmitters for the central nervous system. They carry instructions, as it were, from one cell to another. They could be considered the "hormones" or "messenger chemicals" of the immune system. They enhance or suppress the functions of other immune system cells. Lymphokines also affect other cells and biological functions. In fact, evidence is mounting that lymphokines like interleukin-2 act as chemical bridges between the immune system and the nervous system.

Lymphokines can (and are) classified by researchers in different ways. For example, some are released only in the presence of an antigen, others are not. Different lympho-kines have different target cells. Some are stimulatory, others inhibitory. The best-known lymphokines are inter-leukin-1 and -2, and the *interferons*.

Interferon is the body's most rapidly formed defense against viruses. In fact, it was named "interferon" because it was seen to "interfere" with the ability of viruses to infect the body. At least three kinds of interferon (usually called alpha, beta, and gamma) are known, and a different gene may exist for each one. When interferon is released by a cell in response to stimulation by an invading virus, the compound proceeds to do some stimulating of its own. It causes surrounding cells to release other chemical com-pounds, which in turn may interfere with the virus's ability to multiply, trigger an immune system response, or do other things to inhibit viral infection.

To be a bit more precise, the viral stimulus causes a gene in the cell being attacked to become activated. That gene produces one of several kinds of interferon. The interferon is secreted by the cell into the surrounding fluid. It comes into direct contact with nearby cells. When that happens, genes in their chromosomes become activated and produce various antiviral proteins.

Interferon's ability to trigger the inhibition of the growth of viruses is now well-known and heavily studied. However, interferon also helps to regulate the immune response by its action on various immune cells. Here's one scenario: A foreign antigen of some kind enters the body and comes into contact with an unactivated T cell. That contact causes the T cell to mature and change into an activated T cell. Perhaps it will become a memory T cell, "remembering" that particular antigen in case it ever invades again. Or it may release one or more lymphokines. Interferon is one of the lymphokines produced by such a sensitized T cell. Meanwhile, the antigen has also triggered the growth and maturation of B cells, which in turn produce antibodies against the antigen. The connection between interferons and antibodies is this: All interferons can suppress the different kinds of B and T cells. This suppression of growth and activity becomes less and less effective as T and B cell maturation progresses. Antibody production by an activated B cell—a plasma cell— strongly resists interferon suppression. In this way interferons can act as a modulator of T and B cell action.

However, interferons can also help to enhance the immune response. That's because the protein can and does suppress the action of *suppressor* T cells. The result would be an actual enhancement of the immune response. Also, interferons more effectively inhibit the growth of tumor cells than of normal cells. That suggests a selective anticancer role for interferons. That has led to many exaggerated claims for interferons. However, there is no doubt about the causal relationship between interferon production and a person's natural recovery from viral infections.

Interferons are not the only chemical messengers for the immune system. Interleukin-2 (IL-2) triggers the rapid increase in numbers of T cells, as well as helping their long-term growth. Recently, IL-2 has been getting the same kind of publicity that interferon got in the 1970s. It has also been suffering the same public relations fate. Interleukin-2 does not kill cancer cells itself. Rather, it boosts the growth of T cells like killer Ts, which do kill cancer cells. IL-2 on its own has had very disappointing results in cancer therapy. However, it is showing promise against some cancers under certain carefully controlled conditions. The trick in using the immune system's chemical messengers as effective healing compounds depends on first finding out exactly what they really do in the body, and how and why. It's not an easy task.

The latest "hot" entry in the cancer battle is a lymphokine called *tumor necrosis factor,* or TNF. It appears to be a potent killer of cancer cells, and the biotechnology industry is racing to get a handle on this potential bonanza. Recombinant TNF is already being made and tested in clinical trials on humans. However, researchers are trying to be somewhat cautious in their claims for TNF's effectiveness. They remember too well the hoopla over interferon and interleukin-2.

Said Kamen, "The next big media hype in biotech, I predict, will be immune system chemicals called *colony stimulating factors,* or CSFs. It will be largely hype. But CSFs will in fact be the next serious biotech products." The hype will take place because genetically engineered CSF medicines will have dramatic effects on humans in clinical trials. "But the bottom line," Kamen added, "is that they do work well, and they are relatively safe."

"Colony stimulating factors include interleukin-2, right?" I asked.

Kamen gave me a stern look. "Nothing is an 'interleukin,'" he said. "That's a name invented by a committee and hopefully it will go away. All the interleukins are more accurately called 'hematopoietic growth factors.' Growth factors for blood cells," he added, seeing the look on my face that said "Huh?"

He continued, "Hematopoietic growth factors have potential applications for autoimmune diseases. All blood cells can be categorized into two groups—myeloid cells and lymphoid cells. The immune system cells are the lymphoid cells, as you know—T cells and B cells. Myeloid cells include red blood cells, blood platelets, and also phagocytes—which gobble things up—neutrophils, monocytes, and so on.

"All of the cells in the blood—all of them—are the offspring of the cells in the bone marrow called pluripotent stem cells. And hematopoiesis, the process of blood cell growth and maturation, is regulated by these proteins I'm talking about, the colony-stimulating factors or CSFs. We don't yet know how many CSF chemicals there are. It's probably about ten or so. Yes, interleukin-2 is one, of course. It's responsible for the proliferation of mature T cells. Another CSF is called *erythropoietin*. This factor is involved in the later stages of red blood cell development. It's the hormone in your body that regulates red blood cells, and it's made in the kidneys. Erythropoietin was first discovered in the 1950s. It's been very successful clinically. Amgen, for example, has been doing very well with marketing genetically engineered erythropoietin."

"Now, I understand that the thing with IL-2," I said, "is that to get a therapeutic effect you have to use toxic doses, and if you don't use toxic doses, you don't get a therapeutic effect."

"Well, yeah, but you have to remember that cancer is a difficult problem. By definition, if you want to treat a tumor, you have to kill cells. About a billion of them. GI has kept away from that area until recently. We've been focusing on positive reacting agents, like erythropoietin. There's a clear clinical need for it, and the chances of its working are very high."

Cancer is "a difficult problem," as Kamen put it, because of the very nature of a cancerous cell. It's nothing more than a cell that has *lost its ability to stop growing and multiplying*. Something has damaged its genetic machinery, the commands that stop its growth. So a cancer cell keeps growing. And multiplying. And growing. And multiplying. Tumor cells, carcinomas, are cells that are effectively immortal. At least until they kill the living creature of which they are a part.

As I gathered together the basic information about

cancer, I sometimes found myself reminded of a passage in the New Testament—specifically, a part of Saint Paul's first letter to the early Christian church in Corinth. The human body, Paul says:

> consists not of one member but of many. If the foot were to say, "I am not a hand and so I do not belong to the body," it does not belong to the body any less for that. Or if the ear were to say, "I am not an eye, and so I do not belong to the body," that would not stop its belonging to the body. If the whole body were just an eye, how would there be any hearing? If the whole body were hearing, how would there be any smelling?
>
> As it is, God has put all the separate parts into the body as he [sic] chose. If they were all the same part, how could it be a body? As it is, the parts are many but the body is one. The eye cannot say to the hand, "I have no need of you," nor can the head say to the feet, "I have no need of you."

The immune system was the furthest thing from Saint Paul's mind, of course. He probably didn't know of its existence. But what struck me, as I looked up and read this passage in the *New Jerusalem Bible* translation, was that this could almost be a comment on the relationship between individual cells of the body and the body itself. A cell that has become cancerous and begun multiplying and growing into a tumor is essentially saying to the rest of the body, "I have no need of you. I do not care about you. I care only for myself. I am the center of the universe. I will commandeer all nutrients. *You* feed *me*. Nothing else matters." How can there be any hearing, any smelling, any walking—any living—under these circumstances?

There can't be. The "selfish" tumor is eventually its own downfall. The body finally dies, and so does the tumor. Unfortunately, the body in question is also a human being.

Lunch finished, Bob Kamen talked some about immune system "communication chemicals" that his company was developing for commercial use. One was called GM-CSF, which stands for *granulocyte-macrophage colony stimulating factor*. Said Kamen, "It's a protein thought to be involved in the middle to late stages of the development of the lymphocyte lineages. When we first began working with it, though, no one was quite sure of that. In fact, when we began, GM-CSF it wasn't even clearly defined chemically. So when we started out, we decided to clone and express the gene for GM-CSF. I think that was in 1983. Now we have a product which is licensed to Sandoz, the giant international drug company." When this drug comes on line, it will signal a new way to treat a disease caused by other cancer treatments. It may also help people with AIDS.

The disease caused by some cancer therapies is called *neutropenia*, the loss of the immune system cells known as neutrophils (or granulocytes). Kamen explained: "Neutropenia's caused by bone marrow deficiency or immune suppression, which is a side effect of most cancer drug therapies and of radiation therapy for cancer. The most successful anticancer drugs work by blocking the growth of rapidly proliferating cells."

"And bone marrow cells grow very rapidly indeed."

"Right. Like crazy. So cancer patients have three problems after treatment. They're anemic, they're thrombocytopenic—that is, missing blood platelets—and they're neutropenic. For anemia you transfuse them. For thrombocytopenia you give them packed platelets."

"And for neutropenia?"

"Well, up to now, for neutropenia you put them in intensive care and hope for the best. It's not a *hopeless* situation," added Kamen. "But you can't give people transfusions of granulocytes. Granulocytes are cells that have an extremely short lifetime.

"Neutropenia is bad because neutrophils—granulocytes—are the main defense against bacterial infection. Patients who are neutropenic have a high incidence of those kinds of infection. One of the main roles of granulocyte cells is to keep your blood free of organisms that are abundant in the body—*E. coli,* for example, which is found in the colon and in feces.

"And now, of course, there is AIDS. People with AIDS have bone marrow problems generally. So GM-CSF could be helpful for a serious problem associated with AIDS.

"We are very gratified that GM-CSF appears to do what we thought it would. We are now making it in animal cells on a large scale. Now, one of the complications with in vivo testing of GM-CSF is that it's only active in primates. So we use macaques and other monkeys that are not endangered species.

"And by the way, they're very well treated, they're really pampered. We use rhesus monkeys, too."

The tests Kamen was talking about involved giving test animals doses of GM-CSF and seeing if the numbers of phagocytes—white blood cells—goes up. Normally we have many fewer phagocyte cells in our body than the bone marrow can really produce, since most of them die. When we have an infection, though, there's a great calling up of the troops. Typically in humans the white cell counts are 5,000 to 8,000 per cubic millimeter. A patient with a severe bacterial infection can have a phagocyte count of up to 50,000 to 60,000. Several grams per day of white blood cells are being made in those circumstances.

"We expected that if we gave GM-CSF to an animal—boom—that's what would happen," Kamen told me. "The count would go up to 50,000 or 60,000. In fact, within a few hours of getting GM-CSF there seems to be a release of stored phagocytes. In the most extreme case, we kept a monkey at between 70,000 and 90,000 for four months. And the most amazing thing was, *there were no side effects.* We're in human clinical trials now. I can't talk about the human data, unfortunately, but I can assure you that certainly the monkeys that are being tested are quite well and feel quite well.

"Here's one amazing example of what can be done with GM-CSF," Kamen continued. "We had a young lady monkey that was not making any blood cells at all. She was very debilitated. We used GM-CSF on her for a week, and the animal went from no blood cells to normal. Pow. On the basis of that, Sandoz started a Phase One test of GM-CSF on people with AIDS." Phase One is safety testing. Phase Two is testing for the efficacy, the effectiveness, of a compound. "Now, Sandoz decided to focus on AIDS because we want to see if we can raise these people's white blood cell count. Doing this test in cancer patients would be a bad experiment. The only effective test of this kind would be with terminal cancer patients, and they've already been treated with other things that have failed. So getting a consistent set of data would be very difficult. With people with AIDS, though, you can get a group of people who have not yet been exposed to a whole lot of drugs, and who are often still in relatively good health. So you can get good data."

Of course, the Genetics Institute wasn't the only company working on immune system factors, nor was GM-CSF the only such compound being investigated. "That's true," said Kamen. "For example, the Amgen Corporation has been working on a compound called G-CSF, granulocyte colony stimulating factor. That's a competing product to ours. They're treating cancer patients with it now." Still another one is M-CSF, or macrophage colony stimulating factor. Several biotech companies are working on bringing it to market, also.

Kamen stressed the importance of using factors like GM-CSF in the right way. "Bone marrow transplantation is being used more and more for treatment of some cancers, especially leukemias," he said by way of example. "These people are extremely neutropenic, lasting for three weeks to three months. One way to treat them is with autologous bone marrow transplants. That is, you take some of their own bone marrow out, and store it. Then you kill everything else in their body—the cancer, the bone marrow, and so on. Then you transplant their stored bone marrow back into them. And it works.

"In animal tests, simply using GM-CSF works beautifully to increase the numbers of neutrophils and granulocytes and other blood cells. But with leukemia you can't do this. Leukemia is a cancer of the red blood cells, which are cells that are growth-factor dependent. You do *not* want to give someone GM-CSF to stimulate the growth of their blood cells when they have leukemia! So the idea is to treat the *donor* bone marrow with GM-CSF to increase the number of cells you're going to transplant back into the person."

Kamen and his people at the Genetics Institute aren't stopping with GM-CSF, M-CSF, or G-CSF. They have moved on to still another breakthrough: the discovery of the gene for another human lymphokine dubbed interleukin-3. IL-3 boosts the growth and maturation of lymphocytes at an earlier stage in their growth, before B and T cells have split off from the precursor stem cells in the bone marrow. Other researchers had found the IL-3 gene in mice and rats. In 1986 two Genetics Institute scientists, Steve Clark and Yu-Chung Yang, found a gene in gibbons that was remarkably similar to the mouse IL-3 gene. From there it was a relatively simple step to compare a computerized list of human genes to the gibbon gene, and find one that closely matched it. The human gene in turn produces a chemical that performs the same function in humans that gibbon and mouse IL-3 does in those animals. If clinical trials show that human IL-3 lives up to laboratory tests, this lymphokine could become a major player in the battle against cancer and other illnesses—including AIDS. For example, IL-3 injections might be able to boost the immune systems of AIDS patients, enabling them to battle more effectively against the opportunistic infections that result from AIDS. It might also be used to jump-start the immune systems of cancer patients who have had radiation or chemotherapy for their tumors.

"How long is it going to take you to develop a factor?" I asked.

"It will take us about a year to go from cloning a factor to applying for clinical trial," Kamen replied. "We want to look at four different growth factors: IL-3, GM-CSF, G-CSF, and M-CSF, or macrophage colony stimulating factor. This works on the most mature macrophage cells. We want to use M-CSF to potentiate the growth of monocyte macrophages."

By now it was late in the afternoon. The Genetics Institute was located just a short walk from a Red Line subway station in Cambridge. The trolley would take me straight back, across Boston, to the home where I was staying in Brookline. As I got ready to depart, Robert Kamen left me with words that put his earlier comments in perspective.

"The growth and development of the immune system is really quite exquisite and complex," he said. "And it would be arrogant for anyone to say we understand it."

Growth factors like interleukin-3, GM-CSF, and the others may be the cancer-treating compounds of the future. The hottest and most promising cancer treatment today, though, is with another vital part of the immune system: antibodies. The road to this new cancer treatment stretches back more than eighty years, to 1906.

Paul Ehrlich was two years away from his medicine Nobel. Camillo Golgi and Santiago Ramón y Cajal won the prize that year for their pioneering work on brain cells. Ehrlich, meanwhile, was talking about something that would wander through the fantasies of doctors and immunologists for seventy years. He was speculating about antisera. An antiserum is the serum from the blood of an animal or a human which contains antibodies for at least one antigen. Suppose, said Ehrlich, we could come up with a special kind of antiserum—an antiserum that would not only recognize one kind of cancerous tumor cell, but would actually take part in killing the tumor. This was Ehrlich's idea of a "magic bullet," a biological projectile that would unerringly home in on and destroy one specific target.

Monoclonal antibodies have been called magic bullets, a powerful new method for curing cancer. They certainly could be, and in some cases have already shown remarkable effects. The name itself sounds like science fiction. They are science fact, a reality that is slowly but surely coming to the forefront of medical technology.

Ronald Levy is tall, dark, bearded. His physical presence and personality dominated the room (his office) where we met. Levy works in the Division of Oncology of the Department of Medicine at the Stanford University School of Medicine in Palo Alto, California. He is one of the pioneers and leaders in the field of monoclonal antibody therapy for cancer. I met him on a March afternoon. It was sunny in Palo Alto and windy. The campus, as usual, was beautiful, and I walked around a bit before getting back in my car and driving a circuitous route from the main Stanford campus to the School of Medicine. There was a lot of construction going on—new buildings, roads torn up. I spent long minutes driving slowly through a crowded parking lot looking for an open slot. After I found a spot, I rushed to my appointment. I got lost several times in the maze of corridors, but finally made it to his office. I began our conversation by mentioning an article by him and Dr. James Lowder on the therapeutic and diagnostic uses of monoclonal antibodies against cancer, an article which had been published in December 1985 in the *Western Journal of Medicine*. "Yes, that *was* a pretty good article," said Levy.

"But it was published several years ago, and you and Lowder wrote it even earlier. What's the current direction of the field?" I asked. "Where is monoclonal antibody therapy headed now?"

Levy replied, "I think the main direction the field has moved in is from searching for the good monoclonal antibodies that can distinguish between tumor cells and normal cells, to using them in a way that they can do something therapeutically. On their own monoclonal antibodies don't do too much. They can bind to the tumor cell and focus the immune system on the tumor cell to some degree. But the way in which they kill tumor cells depends on the immune system. The immune system has a limited capacity to do that job.

"The other inherent problem is, the more specific the antibody is, the less comprehensive it gets for the entire tumor population. If you attack the majority of the tumor, that's not enough. You have to attack it all. The problem is that some of the cells in the tumor don't have the target that your antibody sees. Those are the two major limitations of the field.

"So what do you do about it? Well, you incorporate a killing mechanism—such as radioactivity—that can spread beyond the target itself. You can kill a neighboring cell as well as the cell you target. The neighboring cells are caught in the crossfire of radioactive decay."

"So you're talking about using the monoclonal antibodies as a truck carrying in troops if you will, which jump off and attack the enemy."

"Right. But those troops don't have to go inside the cell to work. They work from outside the cell. That's the difference between the radioactive troops and the poison troops. Poisons, like toxins and drugs, have to go inside the cell to work. They will not deal with the problem of the antigen-negative cell. They will only kill the targeted cells more efficiently. The real problem is to kill the nontargeted cell."

Antibodies, of course, are one of the three main active forces of the immune system, along with T cells and nonspecific protective cells. They are the protein molecules made by B cells. Each B cell is unique. When properly stimulated by immune system factors, a B cell will multiply, creating a clone of itself. A clone, in medical terminology, is not an individual but a group of genetically identical individuals. A B cell clone, stimulated into action, produces antibodies, and those antibodies are specific for a unique antigen invader. Different B cells can and do secrete antibodies that react with the same antigen. However, each antibody is still unique. It's just that each "plugs into" a different chemical substructure of the same antigen.

It's pretty easy to make antibodies in the laboratory, either from humans or experimental animals like mice. For example, one can inject a mouse with a specific antigen—a simple, well-known chemical, for example—and the mouse will make antibodies specifically targeted to that antigen. Those antibodies circulate in the mouse's blood, and can be extracted from mouse blood samples. In humans, specific antibodies can be recovered from the blood of individuals who have contracted and recovered from some illness, such as measles or chicken pox.

Ease of production is one thing. Uniformity and quality is another. Remember, each antibody is unique. Even in the case of genetically identical inbred mice, injected with the same chemical, the antibodies will be somewhat different. The billions of potential chemical combinations resulting from the immune system's genetic gene-shuffle ensure that uniqueness. Also, an antiserum containing antibodies specific for a certain antigen also contain lots of other antibodies—kind of a "background antibody noise" that reduces the efficiency and usability of the preferred antibodies for diagnostic or experimental purposes. Another problem: Different animals produce different amounts of an antibody. Some antisera may have only a small amount of an antigen-specific antibody, while other antisera have huge amounts of it. Finally, not all antibodies specific for certain antigen are equally strong. Some may bind very tightly to the antigen in question (good for diagnostics, experiments, and treatment); other antibodies, also specific for the same antibody, may bind to it only weakly.

For years, the production of high quality, highly specific antibodies for medical purposes has been more of an art than a science. The skill and experiment of a researcher— even intuition and hunches—have been as important as any standard technique. Not surprisingly, scientists have long searched for some way to make pure, identical antibodies for research and medical treatment. In the late 1970s that dream came true, with the creation of monoclonal antibodies. They were made possible by two breakthroughs.

The first advance was discovering the actual existence in the body of monoclonal antibodies. That arose from observations made in the 1950s and 1960s of the incredible variety of antibodies. Immunoglobulins, it turned out, were made of thousands of similar yet distinct molecular pieces. What's more, different antibodies coming from different B cells, which bound to the same antigen, *also* were quite variable in structure. These and other observations led researchers to conclude that, first, each B cell and all its progeny makes only one specific, unique antibody. And secondly, the body's population of B cells itself must be incredibly diverse. When an antigen enters the body, it gets exposed to different B cells. Eventually, it meets up with a B cell that bears on its surface a molecular structure that matches some part (or *epitope*) of the antigen. That essentially triggers the B cell to begin dividing into a population of identical cells—a B cell clone, in other words. And each B cell of the clone produces the same antibody. The antibodies are, by definition, *monoclonal antibodies*.

The second breakthrough, fittingly enough for a new tool in the war against cancer, came from the study of a certain cancer. Multiple myeloma is rare, but always fatal. It's a cancer of certain cells in the bone marrow called plasma cells. Plasma cells ordinarily mature into B cells, the producers of antibodies. Victims of multiple myeloma always have huge amounts of immunoglobulin-G in their blood, so much that their blood becomes unusually viscous and "syrupy." When researchers took a closer look, they found that the immunoglobulin proteins in each particular multiple myeloma patient were all identical. These antibodies were not being made to attack some specific invading antigen. They were merely the byproduct of the tumor, gone wild from cancer and pumping out an unending quantity of its particular antibody.

Two researchers in England, Cesar Milstein and Georges Kohler, realized that the medical community had before it two pieces of a puzzle. And that the pieces might fit together into some new kind of pattern. It's very difficult to take a B cell clone that produces a unique antibody and grow it in a test tube. On the other hand, here was a B cell tumor, multiple myeloma, that grew uncontrollably and pumped out plenty of a specific antibody—but an antibody that was useless. Separately, they are nearly useless. But together? Together, Kohler and Milstein realized, the B cell and the tumor cell might make a great team. The B cell would provide the unique antibody. The tumor would supply the ability to grow continuously. In 1975 they announced their success. They had been able to fuse together a myeloma tumor cell with a B cell. The result, a hybrid cell called a *hybridoma,* had the characteristics they were looking for. It was immortal, and produced copious amounts of a specific antibody. Monoclonal antibodies.

Kohler and Milstein's breakthrough revolutionized biology and medicine. (It also won them a Nobel Prize.) It was now possible to make high quality, extremely pure and specific antibody preparations. Standardization became possible. The best and highest quality monoclonal antibodies (eventually abbreviated to MAbs) could be made in virtually inexhaustible amounts. Researchers and doctors could freely exchange samples of their MAbs with others. The variation in quality from lab to lab would be greatly reduced, if not virtually eliminated. But perhaps the greatest advantage of MAbs was the ability to make large quantities of antibodies *targeted on a specific antigen.* Researchers could make MAbs that attacked only certain types of cells. They could even produce MAbs that reacted only with certain *parts* of certain biological molecules. The MAbs would recognize the specific "marker" or "flag" that uniquely distinguishes a cancerous liver cell (for example) from a normal liver cell. The result would be drugs that killed only the cancerous cells, and left the rest of the body unharmed.

To do this, as Levy had mentioned, meant using the MAbs to carry compounds that would actually kill the tumor cells. Radioactive compounds were major contenders. "What kinds would you use with monoclonal antibodies?" I asked Levy.

"There's a great debate now over that," he said. "On the one hand, the universe of radioactive compounds is finite. And on the other hand the chemistry of getting them onto an antibody and keeping the antibody in native form is limited."

Levy noted two kinds of radioactive compounds that cancer researchers are using. "First of all, there are compounds called *alpha emitters*. Their radioactivity kills cells in a very limited area, about one or two cells wide. Then there are *beta emitters* like iodine-131 and yttrium-90. Their energy covers a lot more area, maybe a centimeter. And there are problems with each. It's easier to tie some compounds to monoclonals than others. Iodine is easy, for example. And we've been doing that for a long time. But the iodine is also easily chopped off the monoclonal by certain chemicals in the body. So you often end up getting radioactive iodine coming out in the patient's urine, instead of sticking around near the target cells.

"You have to deal with time limits—delivery time, residence time, cleaving time, elimination time, and the half-life of the isotope, the decay time of the iodine."

"Alpha particles" are the nuclei of helium atoms, two protons and two neutrons bound together. "Beta particles" are nothing more than electrons. An "isotope" is a particular version of an element. Some elements have several versions or isotopes, depending on how many neutrons they have in their nucleus. The half-life of a radioactive element is also a fairly simple kind of thing. "Half-life" is defined as the amount of time it takes for one half of a specific amount of material to decay radioactively from one state to another. After twenty-four hours, 8 ounces of a pound of a radioactive element with a half-life of one day will no longer be radioactive. After another day, half of what's left—4 ounces—will radioactively decay. And so on. In this case, only 1/8 ounce of the original 1 pound will still be radioactive after one week.

Some isotopes have half lives measured in hours or days. Others have half-lives of hundreds of thousands of years.

Most people don't understand half-lives, alpha particles, or beta particles. Radioactivity is radioactivity. It's *evil*. I put the question to Levy: "I can see a problem with the politics of this. There is a general attitude in this country that, if it's radioactive, it's bad. What are you going to do with it? You have to work with compounds with short half-lives, because otherwise you must do something with them after you're finished with them."

Levy nodded. "That's the problem with radioactive compounds that are alpha emitters. They have long half-lives, many years. And you can't detect them easily. They have good tissue-killing properties, short path lengths, but they're hard to detect and not easy to deal with in the safety sense. Now, beta emitters have very good tissue-damaging properties, a longer path length, and have a variety of half-lives. Iodine-131 is about a week. Yttrium-90 has a half-life of about ninety-six hours."

"Iodine's been used for a long time."

"Yes, it's been in medical use for a long time. We have lots of experience in treating thyroid cancer with it. So a lot is known about it."

"Which raises another problem, it seems to me. If the iodine is broken off from the monoclonal antibodies, then it would go—"

"To the thyroid, yes. But that is easily taken care of. You give the person 'cold' iodine in his drinking water. That saturates the thyroid with nonradioactive iodine, and that blocks the uptake of radioactive iodine.

The creation of a particular monoclonal antibody is simple to envision. You find the activated B cell that's making the antibodies you want, and then make a lot of identical copies of the B cell. Simple in theory—but incredibly difficult in practice. It requires sorting through millions of B cells to find just the one you want.

The monoclonal production process begins with the same technique used to make more conventional "polyclonal" antibodies. An experimental animal is immunized against the specific antigen you're interested in dealing with. In the conventional technique, rabbits and goats are used, since they are large and can safely donate substantial amounts of blood. Mice are usually used for the monoclonal technique. Recently, though, some advances have been made in the development of human monoclonal antibodies, based on naturally immunized people. Of course, this would be ideal for MAbs used to treat people. Mouse MAbs are good, but only for a while. Eventually the human immune system identifies the mouse monoclonal antibody as a foreign antigen and mounts an immune response against it. The mouse MAbs then lose their diagnostic or clinical effectiveness.

Up to this point, the old and new antibody technologies are similar. Now things get different. In the conventional method, the animal's serum is the source of the antibody. And it is the result of the production of millions of activated B cells. However, monoclonal antibodies come directly from the B cells themselves. There is no animal serum involved anymore.

A few days after the experimental mouse has been immunized against a particular antigen, it is "sacrificed," i.e., killed. The researchers then remove the mouse's spleen, one of the major organs of the immune system. The mouse spleen is placed in a tissue culture and carefully broken up into millions of individual lymphocytes. Somewhere in the midst of them are the cells of the antibody-making clones that were generated in response to the antigen. The spleen cells are now mixed with myeloma tumor cells in ways that encourage them to fuse with one

The production of monoclonal antibodies

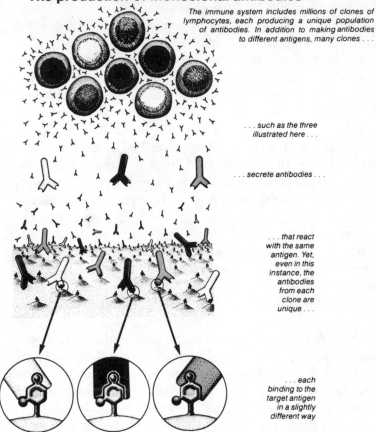

The immune system includes millions of clones of lymphocytes, each producing a unique population of antibodies. In addition to making antibodies to different antigens, many clones . . .

. . . such as the three illustrated here . . .

. . . secrete antibodies . . .

. . . that react with the same antigen. Yet, even in this instance, the antibodies from each clone are unique . . .

. . . each binding to the target antigen in a slightly different way

The production of monoclonal antibodies, shown here in three illustrations, is a long and complex process. Nevertheless, they are now becoming major weapons in the fight against some forms of cancer. *(Illustrations courtesy of the Salk Institute.)*

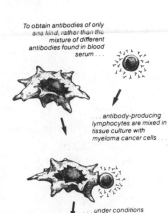

To obtain antibodies of only one kind, rather than the mixture of different antibodies found in blood serum . . .

. . . *antibody-producing lymphocytes are mixed in tissue culture with myeloma cancer cells . . .*

. . . *under conditions favoring cell-cell fusion . . .*

. . . *to yield hybrid cells – hybridomas – that both secrete that lymphocyte's particular antibody and have the endless growth potential of cancer cells.*

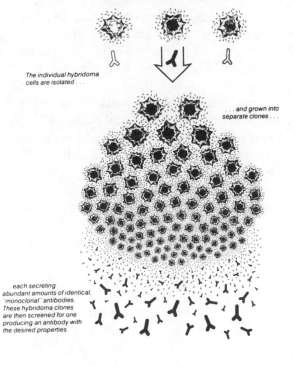

The individual hybridoma cells are isolated . . .

. . . *and grown into separate clones . . .*

. . . *each secreting abundant amounts of identical, "monoclonal" antibodies. These hybridoma clones are then screened for one producing an antibody with the desired properties.*

79

another. Next, chemicals are added to the mixture, which kill the unfused lymphocytes and myeloma cells. Only the hybridomas remain. Each hybridoma now goes into a separate petrie dish, where it is carefully cultured and grown into a clone. Each hybridoma clone happily churns out its own unique brand of antibody.

And now the really tedious part begins. Samples of the fluid from each hybridoma tissue culture are tested to see if they contain the antibody to the target antigen. Thousands, perhaps tens of thousands, of hybridoma cells may result from one mouse spleen. This could take a very long time. Fortunately, microcomputers, sophisticated software, and simple robotic machines make it possible to automate a lot of this testing. The chances of finding the right hybridoma and antibody from one mouse spleen are pretty low. Not all the spleen cells hybridize, not all the spleen cells are antibody-making cells, and most of the ones that do are making the wrong antibody. But with enough time and enough mouse spleens, researchers can make the correct hybridoma and get just the right MAb for their purposes.

The one problem I could see with this whole process of making monoclonal antibodies had to do with mice versus men. "You're using mouse-derived monoclonal antibodies," I said to Levy, "so you have introduced a foreign substance into the body and the immune system will reject it. Shouldn't we be using human monoclonal antibodies?"

"Yes, well . . ." Levy paused. "We are surprisingly slow in generating human monoclonal antibodies."

"Everybody thought that would be the magic bullet," I said.

He shook his head. "What you're talking about now is *not* the major problem," he said. "If it were, we would have solved it. There are other problems. If we could deal with the problem of negative variant cells—cells without the target antigen, and with the problem of good specificity—then the immune reaction problem would be next on the list. I mean, there are ways to take a mouse variable-region gene and hook it to a human constant-region gene and make a chimeric antibody that is mostly human." The constant and variable regions are parts of an antibody molecule. The constant region, as the name suggests, is pretty much the same from antibody to antibody. The variable part of the molecule is not and helps make each antibody clone unique. Levy continued: "The chimeric antibody for human use is about to become available. The Becton Dickinson Corporation in Mountain View, California—not far from here—is making it, and we will use it in a clinical trial next year. This will be the first human test of such antibodies."

A *chimera* (pronounced kye-MEE-rah) is an organism that contains tissue or genes from two genetically distinct "parents." Some science fiction stories speak of creatures made of an amalgamation of chimpanzee genes and human genes. Such a creature (which is at least theoretically possible; there is more genetic variation among humans than between *Homo sapiens* and *Pan troglodytes*) would be a chimera. The word originally refers to the Greek mythical creature that was part lion, part goat, and part serpent. Chimeric plants and animals have already been made. The chimeric antibodies Levy was talking about are made with pieces from two different species, humans and mice. Such antibodies have also been constructed in the laboratory.

Levy and his associates were ready to begin the clinical trials of the new human-mouse chimeric antibodies. The test would involve five to ten cancer patients, and it would last for a year. The results would not be known until the end of 1988. Only then would Levy know for sure if the chimeric monoclonal approach would solve the problem of animal antibodies in humans. "You can deliberately immunize mice," he said. "But you *can't* deliberately immunize humans. That's the main stumbling block. So if you deliberately immunize a mouse, get a mouse hybridoma, and then reengineer it into a human antibody, that may solve this particular problem.

"But—you *still* have to kill the tumor cells efficiently, kill all of them. The immune response against foreign injected proteins is not as important a problem."

I nodded. "A friend of mine died last year of cancer of the liver," I told him. "It had metastasized there from the lungs. She and I were talking with her doctor one afternoon, and he was saying that if they had killed 99.9999 percent of the cancer in the lung, there wouldn't have been any problem. They only got 99.9998 percent of it, and it was that tiny remnant that metastasized."

"That's right," said Levy. "Now, it is obvious that no single method will do the job. At best this will be one to add to all the rest. A mop-up treatment to add to surgery and chemotherapy."

A few days earlier I had been talking with a researcher at the Cetus Corporation in Berkeley. He had been extolling the virtues of polyclonal antibodies versus monoclonal antibodies. I asked Levy about that.

"Polyclonals are a good idea, except they are very hard to make in quantities—unless you have the antigen in large quantities, with which you can purify the polyclonal antibody. In most cases we don't have the antigen. *Something* has to be pure. Either the antibody already has to be pure, or the antigen has to be pure with which you purify the antibody. And if you have that, polyclonals are a good technology. You can make a lot of antibodies. But you are left with the problem of consistency from batch to batch. Every time you immunize your goat, you're going to get a different collection of antibodies."

"Um. Right."

"Whereas if you have a good hybridoma, you've got the same antibody—forever. You just keep milking it. And you can always pool together many different monoclonals and make a custom blend of polyclonals."

"I was wondering if you could do that."

"Oh, sure. Hybridoma technology has gotten very good. We are really addressing the *theoretical* limitations rather than technical limitations.

"So radioactivity is one good way," Levy said briskly, returning to the earlier direction of our conversation. "Another is mixing it with other methods."

"Any ideas in that area? Of mixing?"

"Yes. You're going to see IL-2 a lot, interleukin-2. We know the immune mechanism of killing uses the effector cells. You can amplify the activity of those cells with other biologics, including IL-2 and the interferons. There are many animal experiments that indicate the combinations of antibodies plus interferon or IL-2 are more than additive. There's a synergy between them. There was a recent article in *Science* that reported that using interferon increases the target on the tumor cells and reduces the heterogeneity of the target. Another article showed that interferon actually enhances the killing mechanism of antibodies. And in some diseases these agents have their own therapeutic effects, to which you add the synergistic effects with monoclonal antibodies.

"So that's the other idea you'll be seeing a lot of, the combination of these biologics including antibodies."

"Steven Rosenberg's work at NCI has been rather interesting and controversial, with his LAK cells, lymphokine-activated killer cells. Have you heard anything new?" Rosenberg's work had been front-page news a year earlier. It had even made the nightly television news, with Tom Brokaw of NBC personally reporting the story from

Rosenberg's laboratory. Rosenberg had taken immune cells from patients' blood and incubated them in a bath of interleukin-2. The cells were activated, Rosenberg reported in the December 5, 1985, issue of *New England Journal of Medicine*, and became a form of immune killer cell. He dubbed them "lymphokine-activated killer cells," or LAK cells. He then injected the LAK cells into a number of patients suffering from terminal cancer. The LAK injections were followed by injections of straight IL-2. All other treatments had failed. This was experimental, but perhaps their last chance. The results had been impressive. "A major breakthrough in cancer therapy," the press had trumpeted. Later reports were slightly less effusive. The side effects from the LAK treatment had been very severe. Some of the twenty-five patients in the study gained 20 to 30 pounds of fluid in the first several weeks of therapy. Others suffered serious malfunctions of their liver and kidneys. One patient, Rosenberg reported, died as a direct result of the treatment. Those first experiments had taken place more than a year earlier.

Levy shrugged. "Oh, there's new stuff all the time. Now people are trying to determine whether those cells are actually doing anything at all. Or if it's just the IL-2 that's doing the job."

That surprised me, and I said so.

"Well, the cells are doing something, but what kind of contribution they are making is the question. You can make LAK cells in vivo, in the person, just by injecting IL-2. Whether the additional LAK cells make any difference or not, I don't know.

"But the effects *are* dramatic. You have to admit that. Some of these tumors you never see responses in suddenly have dramatic responses—even though that's not common. There's something in it."

Levy was right about "new stuff all the time." A few

months after our conversation, Rosenberg announced he was using interleukin-2 in a new way. He was taking lymphocytes from pieces of a patient's tumor instead of from his blood. These were immune cells that had been strong enough actually to attack and enter the tumor. Rosenberg was growing these cells in the lab and then soaking them in IL-2 to activate them into what he was calling "tumor-infiltrating lymphocytes"—TILs. He could grow a half pound or more of TILs from an initial sample of a few tenths of an ounce. Animal studies suggested that TIL cells were a hundred times more potent than LAK cells. Early results in humans were also exciting. Tumors in eight of nine patients with melanoma had regressed.

Rosenberg himself was being close-mouthed about it. "The results aren't published," he told one magazine in May of 1988, "and until then I cannot discuss it." But if Rosenberg wouldn't talk about it, others would. Not too surprisingly, the biotech industry had taken Rosenberg's work and was running for the bank. A company called Biotherapeutics, Inc., is using TIL therapy to treat patients referred by their doctors and by the National Cancer Institute. Other companies are collaborating with them in various ways, including biotech giants like Cetus, Amgen, Genentech, and Immunex.

Meanwhile, the monoclonal antibody technology started by Milstein and Kohler is also well on its way to full development. Certainly the possibilities for monoclonal antibodies far exceed Paul Ehrlich's vision of a magic bullet. MAbs are being used in diagnostic tests to monitor the course of a treatment to detect the presence of a disease at extremely early stages. MAbs can be used to detect the minute presence of antigens associated with tumors. And they can be used to treat and perhaps even cure some cancers. Monoclonal antibody treatment for cancer is still not commonplace. It remains experimental for the most part, but the results are pretty good.

Side effects? Sure. Chills and fever are the most common, and people being treated with MAbs sometimes also experience nausea, vomiting, diarrhea, facial edema (their faces swell with water in the tissue), and occasionally a drop in blood pressure. The most common way of relieving the side effects is to stop the monoclonal antibody injections temporarily. Despite the side effects, the treatments continue. They're worth the suffering, because the trade-off is life.

Most of the clinical trials of MAbs for cancer treatment have been against leukemia or lymphomas. Most people know what leukemia is: a cancer of the red blood cells. Thirty years ago, childhood leukemia was a major killer of youngsters. A fourth-grade classmate of mine, in fact, died of leukemia. Today childhood leukemia is not the killer it was back then. The vast majority of youngsters afflicted with it are cured. Adults contracting leukemia aren't so well-off. So much work still needs to be done.

Not so many people are familiar with lymphomas. Lymphomas are cancers of the cells associated with the lymphatic system. Hodgkin's disease is one well-known lymphoma. It begins in the lymph nodes. Researchers now believe that most lymphomas connected with the lymph nodes are B cell or T cell malignancies. Burkitt's lymphoma is a cancer of B cells and stem cells, which are the precursors to most of the lymphatic and immune systems' cells. At least a few lymphomas are caused by viruses. Burkitt's lymphoma has been associated with the presence of the Epstein-Barr virus. One form of T cell lymphoma is caused by the HTLV-I virus, discovered by Robert Gallo.

Levy and his associates were working mainly with B cell lymphomas, he told me, though T cell lymphomas are also treatable with monoclonal antibodies. The reason for working with the B cell cancers, he added, is that they know the target.

"We know the molecules on the surface of B cell tumors that the monoclonal antibody can recognize," said Levy. "We know less about those kinds of things on other kinds of cancer cells and other cells in the body. There, it is a little more hit-and-miss. But there's been a lot of hitting and missing going on. Over the last few years we've been able to find out which antibodies are really the best ones for monoclonal treatments."

The ideal MAb for cancer treatment would be an antibody that could "see" some unique target on a tumor cell, some molecular structure that only appeared on cancerous cells and on nothing else in the body. Such a target *may* exist—but at this point there is no antibody known that could find it. But, in this case, second best is still pretty good, said Levy. "There are quite a few monoclonal antibodies that react with substances restricted to tissue types represented by the tumor. So, for example, we know about the target molecules on colon cancer, melanoma, renal cell cancer, and lung cancer. We know which monoclonal antibodies can recognize them in a relatively restricted way. That's good enough for therapy, good enough so that if the monoclonal antibodies were potent killers, they would add a lot to our therapies."

Levy smiled. "Here's something that is interesting, by the way. The very tumors that occasionally show spontaneous regressions—that sometimes just disappear on their own, for no known reason—those are the ones that IL-2 and LAK cells work on, that interferon works on, and that monoclonal antibodies work on." Levy leaned forward over his desk. "There is a recurring theme here," he said. "This is no accident."

Levy was implying that so-called spontaneous regressions were actually caused by the immune system—a startling comment. Perhaps the body's own supply of interferon and interleukin-2 was, unknown to physicians, attacking and killing the tumor. Later, listening to this part of the tape of our conversation, I would think of Lourdes and of "inexplicable cures" dubbed miracles. A miracle, of course, is by definition something with no *known* explanation. Miracle cures can be—and often are—simply cures for which the contemporary medical community had (or has) no known explanation. Sometimes "demonic possession" turns out to be schizophrenia. Sometimes miraculous cancer cures turn out to be spontaneous regressions triggered by the body's own armies of interferon, interleukin-2, or LAK cells.

I changed the subject. "What about using monoclonal antibodies for imaging tumors inside the body?"

Levy shook his head. "I don't think it will ever work. I don't think imaging is in the cards for antibodies. They don't concentrate at the site of tumors that much. Other imaging technologies, like nuclear magnetic resonance, or CT scans, or imaging using a potent biologic sponge pulling in the radioactive isotope, those are really valuable diagnostic tools. But monoclonal antibodies will never be that. You'll hear a lot of people say they will, but I don't think so."

Levy's eyes twinkled. "So I'm negative on imaging, negative on immunotoxins. And positive on radioactive antibodies and positive on combinations of biologics!" We both laughed.

"How about diagnostic tests with monoclonals?"

"Oh, we use them now, of course. For example, our pathology department here rarely makes a diagnosis without using an antibody test. It's really revolutionized pathology. It's incredible. The predictions of that a few years ago have all come true. I mean, there are antibodies on the shelf that help the pathologist tell the difference between a B cell and a T cell and a lymphocyte and a nonlymphocyte. And beyond that, between a liver cell and a kidney cell. So when they see a tumor—"

"Boom."

"—they can figure it out. Yes. Some of this is already available in your doctor's office. Pregnancy testing, allergy testing, thyroid function testing, hormone measurements. Well, maybe not in your doctor's office, but certainly in the lab he sends his stuff to down the street. Monoclonal technology is replacing all the old tests and creating a lot of new tests."

"How far in the future are some of these new treatments you've hinted at? Are we really close to seeing this become very common?"

"Diagnostic use? That's permeating everything. More and more all the time. Treatments? I think that will be a while, another five years at least."

"Before I can walk into my doctor's office and get weekly treatments."

"Antibody-based treatments, yes. I think we are still trying to figure out how to make it work. Once we do that, it will get around fast. The lag time for a treatment shown to be effective and to become available is pretty low. There are some regulatory barriers and some educational barriers, but I think the real problem is making it work. We are still not quite there yet."

One of Levy's recent articles had described the molecular structure of the CD4 molecule, the receptor on the T4 cell used by the AIDS virus as its "gateway" into the cell. "I think it's all well and good that we've figured out the molecular structure of the molecule," I said. "But I know people, friends of mine, who will ask why that's necessary. Why spend the time and money on something esoteric like that? What's the point?"

"Why do we need to know the characteristic of the CD4 molecule?" said Levy. "Well, we really didn't know how AIDS got into the cell *until* we knew about CD4 molecule. And it was discovered with a monoclonal antibody. We didn't know its existence until a monoclonal antibody was discovered that divided T cells into different groups. They had different functions. And people wanted to know what molecules determined these functions. When people discovered AIDS, they realized that it infects only one of the different kinds of T cells, and uses the CD4 molecule as the receptor for the virus.

"That is an amazing concordance of scientific observation," he said. "That's how progress gets made. People don't know in advance why some things are important. So it is critically important that we know something about the molecule, the things that determine function and interaction with cells. Why do basic research? This is a great example of how basic research pays off. We are miles ahead now from where we were. We have cells we can infect, receptors we can go after. A whole therapeutic strategy is based on blocking the receptor for the AIDS virus. Knowing the structure of the CD4 molecule, we can make dummy molecules to distract the virus."

"Is there a strategy here for a vaccine with decoys?"

"Yes! One whole idea for making a phony molecule, a decoy, is to induce one. This is complicated, but the immune network has antibodies against antibodies against antibodies. OK?"

"They're called idiotypes and anti-idiotypes, if I recall correctly," I said. An *idiotype* is an antigenic pattern which the immune system detects and to which it reacts. An *anti-idiotype* is a pattern that is the mirror image of an idiotype. The concept of idiotypes was first developed by Niels Jerne to provide an explanation of how the immune system works. Jerne won the Nobel Prize for his idiotype theory—but some molecular biologists and immunologists are still not too sure how "real life" it is.

"Right. So that if you take the CD4 molecule and have an antibody against it, and use *that* as a vaccine, the body will make an anti-anti-CD4, which will mimic the CD4, and that will occupy the attention of the AIDS virus. That's one whole strategy."

"Is it possible to make large quantities of CD4 molecules?"

"It's possible to make large quantities of anti-CD4 molecules, and anti-anti-CD4 molecules."

"Which in turn mimic the CD4 molecule?"

"Right," Levy said, and went on to offer an example. Suppose you have found an antibody that can tell the difference between a tumor cell and a normal cell. However, you still don't know what exact antigen that antibody attacks. You don't know its exact target. Indeed, said Levy, this is not an uncommon situation with cancer patients. Now, though, it is possible to take the known antibody and use it as a mold to induce the creation of a second antibody, which in turn, is an internal image of the antigen. That second antibody is the anti-idiotype antibody. It acts against the original antibody. Part of that original antibody fits into the tumor antigen. But parts of the original antibody and the second antibody also fit together. The part of the second antibody (the anti-idiotype antibody) that fits that part of the original antibody must therefore be very similar to the antigen.

Now you can use the anti-idiotype antibody (the second antibody) to induce an immune response. To the immune system, the anti-idiotype antibody looks like the antigen; therefore you can induce an immune response against the tumor. These anti-idiotype antibodies can thus be used to make a vaccine that induces the immune system to attack the tumor cells, even though the exact antigen remains unknown.

"Are you people working on that?" I asked.

"Yes. That's another whole way to go," said Levy. "So you can add that to the list of things I'm positive on."

"How far away are you from vaccines?"

"We start our first trials this summer [1987] with an idiotype vaccine against lymphoma."

As with the genetic shuffling mechanisms that create antibody diversity, the use of anti-idiotype antibodies had a certain amount of elegance to it. I said so to Levy, and remarked that the elegance of the "internal image" description made it sound like it *had* to work. "It's sort of like physicists," I said, repeating the comments I had made to Lee Hood. "Physicists and mathematicians are into elegance and beauty in their equations, too. Of course, sometimes it doesn't work."

Levy nodded. "Yes, you have to put it in the real world to make it compete with other things.

"In the end, you have to put it into people with cancer."

4 Autoimmune Diseases— the Turncoats

The body's immune system is supposed to be able to tell the difference between Self and Not Self. That's the essence of its operation. Sometimes, though, that operation goes awry. The body turns against itself. It's called *autoimmunity*, and it results in the appearance of *autoimmune diseases*. More than forty such conditions have been identified so far. They range from such well-known illnesses as Type I diabetes, multiple sclerosis, myasthenia gravis, lupus, and rheumatoid arthritis, to obscure afflictions such as glomerulonephritis, hemolytic anemia, and scleroderma.

For quite some time, many researchers have believed that the susceptibility for certain autoimmune diseases is genetically determined. The diseases in this category include Type I diabetes and rheumatoid arthritis (abbreviated RA). About 50 percent of the identical twins of

93

diabetic patients, for example, eventually develope Type I diabetes. Data on rheumatoid arthritis is not as good as that on Type I diabetes, but it's estimated that 40 to 50 percent of all identical twins come down with it, too. The people with the highest risk of coming down with Type I diabetes have a specific and rather uncommon collection of genes. In one survey of twenty-four families with 107 members, researchers found that all of the siblings with this somewhat rare genetic collection had Type I diabetes. Another survey of families included in its members sixty-six cases in which two siblings had juvenile rheumatoid arthritis. This study showed a definite correlation between having the illness and having this unusual collection of genes. The genetic association for susceptibility to these diseases is connected to the region in chromosome 6 that codes for the immune system. The area is generally called the MHC, or major histocompatibility complex. In humans this part of the chromosome is called the HLA region.

Until recently, there has not been much that anyone could do for someone afflicted with an autoimmune disease except try to alleviate the symptoms. Now the picture is beginning to change, thanks to advances in genetics, molecular biology, and immunology. Researchers are beginning to discover what causes specific autoimmune diseases and how to cure them. For those diseases that may not yet have cures, there are new and effective treatments of the symptoms that are making life worth living again for tens of thousands of people. Three groups of researchers, in particular, have played significant roles in elucidating the genetic connections for Type I diabetes and juvenile rheumatoid arthritis. They include two scientists at Harvard University, two at Stanford University—and a husband-and-wife team at the Virginia Mason Medical Center in Seattle, Washington: Gerald and Barbara Nepom. Their findings are now moving out of the laboratory and into commercial use.

Jerry Nepom's laboratory and office was in an older-looking building across the street from the Virginia Mason Medical Center. A few blocks away was Interstate 5, the main north-south freeway corridor of the west coast. I-5 runs from just north of Tijuana, Mexico, to the Washington-Canadian border. On any given day, at least one part of this superhighway is under reconstruction, revision, or repaving. Where it runs through Seattle, however, I-5 is basically untouched. It was the *city* that was under reconstruction. A huge convention center was being built *over the freeway*. On the other side of I-5 from Nepom's office, Seattle's main downtown area was being dug up to construct an underground bus tunnel. Getting into, through, or around Seattle was a major accomplishment. Despite my familiarity with Seattle—I frequently come up from my home sixty miles to the south—I had difficulty getting to Nepom's side of town. Once there, I struggled to find a parking place before climbing up two flights of stairs to his laboratory.

Nepom's office was crowded with journals and books, but also had its occupant's own sense of order. Nepom himself was of medium height, with a mustache, dark hair, and piercing eyes. His voice was soft, almost melodic.

Jerry Nepom is one of this country's acknowledged experts in the field of autoimmune diseases—illnesses caused when the body's immune system attacks some part of the body itself. In particular, his work has focused on two autoimmune illnesses. One is Type I diabetes, also called juvenile-onset diabetes and insulin-dependent diabetes mellitus or IDDM. The other is a form of rheumatoid arthritis that attacks youngsters, called juvenile rheumatoid arthritis. I had first come across his name in an article in the Seattle *Times* about his work on Type I diabetes. The news media had seen an article by Nepom in a medical journal and pounced on a good story. What I was first interested in, though, was Nepom himself. Once we both settled in, I asked him about history.

"How'd you end up here at Virginia Mason?" I began. "You've apparently gone from one place to the next, before ending up here."

Nepom nodded. "Yeah, it has been an interesting circuit. I got my M.D. and Ph.D. here in Seattle. I was an undergraduate at Harvard when a mentor of mine told me of the Hellstroms who were here in Seattle. I came out here to do my Ph.D. with them, and also got my M.D. at the University of Washington. Then I went back to Harvard for my postdoc and fellowship years. I became an instructor at the Harvard Medical school, working with Baruj Benacerraf. He got the 1980 medical Nobel Prize for his pioneering work in immunogenetics. He, George Snell, and Jean Dausset shared the Nobel that year. Benacerraf was the immunologist, Snell was the mouse geneticist, and Dausset was the human geneticist. It was a tripartite approach to discovering the immune response genes. My training in his laboratory was based on the mouse, to learn how the immune response genes function. So I got some good training in how the immune genes in the mouse work.

"As a result of that, I started thinking about the rest of my life. I ended up moving back here to Seattle where both my wife and I had good offers. I joined the Fred Hutchinson Cancer Center in 1981, and Barbara joined the staff of Children's Hospital as a pediatric rheumatologist and worked in my laboratory. That went along very well for two and a half to three years. Finally I left and joined Genetic Systems Corporation here in Seattle, and set up an immunogenetics program over there.

"I should mention that part of my transition from Harvard to Seattle was a transition from mouse to man."

"Lee Hood told me, when I was talking with him earlier, that he spends, at the most, a third of his time involved with the work of his lab. And at least that much time just involved in running the Biology division at Cal Tech."

Nepom nodded. "Yeah, I believe it. That's why this is really an ideal setup," he said. "There are no departments and no heavy-duty bureaucracy. I'm pretty free to run things the way I want. There's a lot of flexibility, and not a massive amount of paperwork. It's a pretty good deal." Comfortable and challenged at the same time, Nepom had proceeded to make some significant breakthroughs in the field of autoimmune diseases.

Knowing what causes an autoimmune reaction, and thus an autoimmune disease, begins with knowing how the immune system normally works. Lee Hood, John Farrar, Robert Kamen, and others had laid out those basics for me during my visits with them. The main parts of the immune system—the humoral, the cellular, and the nonspecific immune responses—work sequentially and synergistically to recognize, attack, and destroy invading antigens. Macrophage cells, part of the nonspecific arm of the immune system, begin by gobbling up a foreign substance. They chop it up and then "present" pieces of the substance proteins out onto their surfaces. They do this by placing these protein fragments into grooves in the HLA Self-marker molecules on their surfaces.

Along come some T cells, which "see" the antigen fragments nestled in the HLA molecules' grooves. They recognize them as foreign, and as being associated with a Self-marker molecule. It's the process of MHC restriction at work. The T cell now "knows" that a Self cell is infected with an invading antigen. That triggers the cellular immune response.

The activated T cells begin secreting various immune system chemicals. Some of the chemicals trigger certain B cells to change into plasma B cells and secrete antibodies, the specific "bullets" aimed at particular antigens. Still other immune system chemicals—such as interleukin-2—trigger the activation of the cytotoxic or killer T cells. These T cells attack and destroy invaders like viruses.

When the invading antigens are all inactivated or destroyed, suppressor T cells move in to slow down and stop the immune response. Interleukin-2 receptors on killer T cells shrivel and disappear. The killer Ts stop killing. What's left, finally, are "memory" immune cells—T cells and antibodies circulating through the bloodstream and the lymph system, carrying a molecular memory of the antigens that first caused the problem. If those invaders should ever reappear, the immune system will again swing into action. This time, though, the presence of the memory cells will assure a much swifter immune response.

That's what's *supposed* to happen. And if the immune system functioned perfectly all the time, people like Jerry Nepom would be in some other line of work. But it doesn't. The immune system is *not* supposed to attack the body itself. Each T cell can recognize a specific antigen that's nestled in the HLA molecule's groove. However, in the normal course of events, there should exist few if any T cells that would recognize fragments of a person's own proteins. Those self-reacting T cells are destroyed before they reach maturity. Most immunologists think this happens in the thymus, where T cells grow to maturity. How that happens is really not understood, and remains one of the great puzzles of immunology. In laboratories around the world, researchers are racing to find the answer to that question. The first ones to come up with the solution have a big medal and a lot of cash waiting for them in Stockholm.

Sometimes, though, what isn't supposed to happen, does. A person with an autoimmune disease has T cells that attack his or her own bodily proteins. The specific cells involved differ from disease to disease, but the essential process is the same.

Consider Type I diabetes, the focus of much of Nepom's research. The scene of the action is the pancreas, the organ in the body that produces insulin. Insulin is a hormone that is secreted by cells called beta (or β) cells, which are found in a part of the pancreas called the islets of Langerhans. Insulin is essential for the body's proper use of glucose or blood sugar. Too much insulin, and your glucose levels drop disastrously. You end up with extreme hypoglycemia and go into insulin shock. Not enough insulin, and you end up with diabetes, which is characterized by hyperglycemia (excessive glucose).

Type I diabetes is a specific form of diabetes that usually shows up in people younger than twenty-five years. Its appearance is sudden; there is rarely any kind of chemical or medical symptoms that signal its imminence. It's characterized by a nearly total loss of the ability of the pancreas to produce insulin. Thus the person's blood has little or no insulin. In contrast, adult-onset diabetes usually begins gradually and doesn't appear until after forty years of age. There is usually still some insulin in the bloodstream of people with adult-onset diabetes. For them, the symptoms can usually be controlled with proper diet. Some people with adult diabetes also need to take regular doses of insulin. For those with Type I diabetes, however, the only way to control the progress of the disease is with regular insulin injections. Adult diabetes is usually stable and easy to control. Type I diabetes is not. It's a tough companion to go through life with, and there is no cure.

Firm evidence now exists that Type I diabetes is an autoimmune disease with a clear genetic linkage. It begins when something—perhaps a virus—attacks and damages cells in the pancreas. Appropriately enough, macrophages of the immune system ingest the damaged cells and present fragments of proteins in their HLA markers. Some of the protein fragments that end up in the grooves of the HLA markers are pieces of pancreatic β cells. Normally, the immune system's T cells would ignore these fragments. Some people, though, have a genetic susceptibility for Type I diabetes. In these people the HLA markers are slightly different. They bind and present different pieces of pancreas proteins than do the HLA molecules in people without the genetic tendency. Their T cells do *not* recognize these fragments as part of the body. They see them as foreign antigens. The immune system is activated, and in this case it is against part of its own body. Killer T cells attack and begin destroying the β cells of the pancreas. The final result: Type I diabetes.

This new understanding of Type I diabetes fits well with an old observation. Researchers have known for some time that there is an association between the likelihood of getting some autoimmune diseases, and the presence of particular kinds of HLA molecules. One type of HLA molecule seems to be associated with, say, Type I diabetes. Another kind is connected to the likelihood of coming down with multiple sclerosis, and still another with susceptibility for rheumatoid arthritis. In fact, we know that there are millions of possible HLA molecules, and each person carries eight different types on his or her cells.

Two key discoveries have revolutionized our understanding of autoimmune disease. One is in the realm of molecular biology, the other in the field of genetics. In the fall of 1987, two researchers at Harvard announced that they had finally been able to figure out the actual physical structure of the HLA molecule from a human cell. Three thousand miles away in Seattle, Jerry Nepom was pinpointing the precise locations of HLA genes that are connected with susceptibility for Type I diabetes and juvenile rheumatoid arthritis.

The two Harvard researchers, Jack Strominger and Donald Wiley, first made crystals of a human HLA molecule. Then they used X rays to figure out the structure of the molecule. The process is called X-ray crystallography. An early, crude version of this technique led to the discovery of the structure of the DNA molecule in the early 1950s by Francis Crick, James Watson, and Maurice Wilkins. The painstakingly constructed X-ray pictures of the HLA molecule showed that it had a long groove. That groove is the location where specific protein fragments become bound to the HLA molecule, making the MHC-restriction process possible. With this structural information of one HLA molecule finally available, researchers can figure out the shapes of others. The picture put together by Strominger and Wiley is a kind of Rosetta Stone. Researchers now know both the chemical and physical structure of one HLA molecule—the Rosetta Stone molecule. They also know, or can figure out, the chemical structure of other HLA molecules. By comparing these with the Rosetta Stone HLA molecule, they can come up with a rough but reasonably accurate idea of their physical structures.

That, in turn, means researchers will have a better handle on exactly how and why specific antigenic protein fragments fit into specific HLA molecular markers. It also means they can make some good guesses at which drugs might fill up and block the grooves of HLA molecules—specifically the HLA molecules that are involved with autoimmune reactions. That will lead to the development of drugs that would prevent those HLA molecules from triggering an autoimmune reaction in the first place—in other words, cures for autoimmune diseases. Such drugs would not cripple the immune system, either. Each cell carries eight different HLA markers. A drug specifically designed to block the action of the one involved in an autoimmune reaction would not clog up the others.

The next step will be the identification of the specific HLA molecule markers associated with particular auto-immune diseases—the multiple sclerosis HLA molecule, for example, or the Type I diabetes HLA molecule, and so on. That kind of information would lead to diagnostic tests that would identify people at risk for those diseases. Then it would be possible to treat them with immune-suppressing drugs at the very first sign of illness.

Nepom's work at Virginia Mason will provide still another route to diagnostic tests for autoimmune diseases. Over the last several years Nepom and his colleagues have clearly defined the genetic linkage for Type I diabetes and juvenile rheumatoid arthritis. While Strominger and Wiley have come at autoimmune diseases from the angle of molecular biology, Nepom and his team have taken the genetic route. Nepom's findings are so detailed, in fact, that they can already be used to develop diagnostic tests. Tests for genetic predispositions to certain diseases already exist. For example, it's possible to test the amniotic fluid from a pregnant woman and find out if her unborn child is afflicted with certain genetically caused diseases. Tests based on Nepom's findings would be similar. Those tests could also be given to children whose families have a history of Type I diabetes. The family doctor would be able to tell if a particular child had the HLA markers that are typical of people who come down with the disease.

The research being carried out by Nepom and his lab has three main branches. First of all, there is clinical research, including a predictive study of the tendency toward juvenile rheumatoid arthritis, which involves about three hundred people. Nepom is also interested in learning the origin of the different genes involved in the tendency toward juvenile rheumatoid arthritis and Type I diabetes. This is a study which he's doing in collaboration with Leroy Hood at Cal Tech. The third branch of Nepom's research is in the area of regulation. "How exactly are these genes expressed?" he asks. "How do they 'turn on'?"

Finding the answer to the origin of the juvenile rheumatoid arthritis and Type I diabetes genes will be intellectually satisfying. The results of his predictive juvenile rheumatoid arthritis study will fine-tune the ability of doctors to predict who is most likely to come down with this form of rheumatoid arthritis. The answers to the third big question—how do the juvenile rheumatoid arthritis and Type I diabetes genes turn on—will be a tremendous medical breakthrough with dramatic consequences for thousands—perhaps millions—of people.

"Our work on juvenile rheumatoid arthritis is what we're mainly known for," said Nepom. "But this paper in *Lancet* [on Type I diabetes] just came out. It's not so well known, but judging from the numbers of calls we've had from people who want the probe, it will be well known."

"Was the news media interest a surprise?" I asked.

Nepom replied, "Actually, it was. I knew that *Lancet* and the *New England Journal of Medicine* are picked up by some news services, so I wasn't totally surprised. I guess what surprised me was the extent of it. It went out on the AP and UPI wires and was picked up by little town newspapers all around. I've been getting all kinds of interesting calls and letters. It's been kind of fun." He chuckled. "I'm sure that you'll appreciate that some people walk the publicity line very well. Lee Hood is a master at it. It's important to communicate with the public what you're doing, so the public knows that science is not just, you know, mad scientists running around torturing little pink bunny rabbits or whatever. Or doing things that get Golden Fleece Awards from Senator Proxmire. I think we have an obligation to communicate to the public what science *really* is. On the other hand, you can easily go too far and become too far out—talking about yourself, you know—and cross that line."

"Become too self-serving?"

"Yeah. Right. I think that's a line that we should all be aware of.

"It's a little easier here, to walk that line," he added. "Seattle is out of the limelight. I've often said that, if I were doing the same work in my old lab at Harvard, this would be front-page stuff. And I think there's a certain aspect of being here, that that attention takes longer to arrive. But also, I don't have to worry about that stuff."

Nepom, Wiley, and Strominger aren't the only people looking at the genetic tendency toward Type I diabetes. In October 1987, three researchers from Stanford University announced a dramatic finding in just that area. John Todd, John Bell, and Hugh McDevitt traced a major part of the genetic predisposition for the disease to a particular part of the HLA complex. Even more dramatically, they pinpointed a specific single change in one "genetic word," which all by itself greatly increased the chances of a person getting Type I diabetes.

The HLA complex on human chromosome 6 encodes three different classes of genes called, predictably, classes I, II, and III. The class I genes code for the transplantation antigens that appear on every cell of the body. The class III genes are genes that code for the complement proteins of the immune system, which amplify the immune response. The class II genes encode the HLA molecules found on T cells and other immune system cells. These are the ones that would be involved in an autoimmune response. It's the HLA molecules on macrophages, for example, that present pancreas protein fragments to T cells as if they were foreign antigens.

There are quite a few class II gene groups. Each gene group has its own variations and subgroups. More than half of the inherited predisposition to Type I diabetes can be traced to the HLA complex. Todd, Bell, and McDevitt were interested in a particular region of the HLA complex. It runs from the so-called HLA-DR1 genes to the ones called the DRw14 genes. Even more specifically, analysis of DNA sequences in Type I diabetes patients show that different *alleles* of the HLA genes in the HLA-DQ-β region determine both resistance to Type I diabetes and susceptibility for it. An allele (pronounced either "uh-LEEL" or "uh-LEL," take your pick) is one of two or more different genes, which carry the genetic code for a specific inheritable characteristic. Allelic genes occupy corresponding positions on paired chromosomes. Remember: chromosomes come in pairs. Those positions geneticists refer to as *loci* (pronounced "LO-seye"). A collection of allelic genes in a specific area of a chromosome is called a *haplotype*. The prefix *haplo-* comes from the Greek word *haploos*, meaning "single, simple" as opposed to "complex."

The Stanford researchers found that a particular haplotype in the HLA called HLA-DR4 was very closely associated with the likelihood of getting Type I diabetes. The molecules that are encoded by the genes called DR-α and DR-β-1 come together to make a glycoprotein that sits on the surface of an immune cell, such as a T cell. The glycoprotein is called *heterodimeric* by chemists and biologists. A *dimer* in chemistry is a molecule made of two identical simple molecules, or a chemical compound made of such molecules. *Di-* is a Greek prefix meaning "two" or "doubled," and *-mer* comes from the Greek word *meros*, meaning "part." Thus, "two parts." The prefix *hetero,* of course, means "other"; it's used to indicate dissimilar parts, pieces, people, sexes, or whatever. So a protein that is a "heterodimer" is one that's made of two identical parts, but that comes in many dissimilar versions. That describes the HLA cell-surface markers to a *T.* Each such cell-surface glycoprotein is made of two polypeptide chains called "alpha" (α) and "beta" (β). The chains are, ideally, identical. But there are hundreds of millions—perhaps billions—of unique HLA glycoprotein molecules, one for each unique person.

The story didn't end with DR4 alleles. Todd, Bell, and McDevitt found two alleles in the DQ haplotype region that seemed to have a significant connection with the DR4 region in people with Type I diabetes. Those genes are called DQw3.2 and DQw3.1. The former is to be found in as many as 95 percent of all Type I diabetes patients who also have the DR4 genetic grouping. Only 60 to 65 percent of normal people who had the DR4 haplotype also had the DQw3.2 gene. The DQw3.1 gene, on the other hand, had either neutral or negative associations with Type I diabetes. That is, if this gene were present, the person was quite likely *not* to have juvenile diabetes. The researchers then looked at the two protein chains of the molecules that were encoded by these genes. They wanted to find out if there were any differences in the amino acids between the two protein chains. Such differences would mean changes in the proteins. That in turn might well be the cause of a person's high susceptibility to Type I diabetes.

What they found confirmed this hypothesis. There were four places in the DQw3.1 molecular chain with amino acids different from those in DQw3.2. One difference was very important, the amino acid in position 57 in the protein. If the amino acid in that position was asparagine, the person was almost certain *not* to suffer from juvenile diabetes. The *presence* of asparagine in that particular position in that particular molecular chain appears to confer immunity to Type I diabetes.

On the other hand, if *any other* amino acid occupies that particular position in the β chain of that particular HLA marker protein, the structure of the molecule is changed. That makes it extremely likely that a person *will* have the autoimmune reactions that eventually destroy the pancreas's islet cells, and thus cause Type I diabetes.

The work by Todd, Bell, and McDevitt dovetailed nicely with Nepom's. They were different pieces of the same puzzle, and the puzzle was being solved.

But work on any huge jigsaw puzzle can get tedious and tiring, whether it's one on a living room card table or in a laboratory at Stanford. Or a lab in Seattle. During one of my visits with Nepom, as we got ready to take a quick tour of his laboratory area, I asked him how he avoided burning out from the mixture of tedium, boredom, and stress that confronts all serious scientific researchers.

Nepom nodded. "I finally figured out the solution to that. I borrowed it from my old mentor, Baruj Benacerraf. Every August he would basically can the lab. Shut it down." I laughed appreciatively. "Yeah," he continued. "He'd go to his place on Cape Cod. And I finally figured out why he did that. It was for his own sanity. And that's what I'm doing. I've asked everybody to bunch their vacations in August. And this is the first week when it's really worked. So basically the lab is very quiet, because everyone's gone. And I'm finally going to be able to more or less get on top of the paperwork. Then next week I'm going to take a vacation, which will be a nice treat."

"Where are you going to go?"

"Oh, probably we'll just go out to the coast for a few days, to Neah Bay."

"So, it's quiet this morning."

"Yeah. Pretty quiet. Some people will be here working, but they aren't in yet." Nepom paused. "Basically what I try to do, to keep things running smoothly, is I try to make the mornings the time when I'm available to people. That's really effective."

I nodded. "Do you wander about, or just stay here in the office and be available?"

"No, no, I wander about, and check in with everybody. Some days I don't make it through everybody, but I make up for it the next day. My personal philosophy is that if you really want to be a functioning scientist, you have to keep your lab small enough to do that. That's what I've got here. It's a lab of about eighteen people. That's a good size for that kind of thing. I'm able to keep my hand in the work a little.

"The last few months have been marvelous. We've gotten a few more people in. Got a few more grants. Starting next Monday we're renovating another 2,500 square feet down the hall here. That's the rest of this floor. So things are working out very nicely. I feel like this is a little . . . Mecca or whatever the word is—a refuge, I guess."

Nepom smiled his slight, barely impish smile. "You'll appreciate this, because you know Lee Hood. Well, we just recruited someone from his lab. We feel good about that recruitment, because this guy had a number of good offers from what most people consider more prestigious labs. But he chose to come here.

"You realize," he explained, "we've only been here a little more than a year, since January of 1986. I came from a lab at Genetic Systems where I had six or seven people. Here at Virginia Mason I have sixteen or seventeen people now."

One of the newest staff members in Nepom's lab was his wife Barbara. She had been at Children's Hospital, but had gotten a five-year NIH research grant to continue her work on juvenile rheumatoid arthritis. Children's didn't have the kinds of facilities that Barbara Nepom needed for her project, so she had filed her grant application through Jerry's lab. Getting the grant meant doing her project at Virginia Mason instead of Children's. Her primary appointment was still at Children's Hospital, but Virginia Mason also gave her an appointment as an affiliate investigator in her husband's laboratory. At the time I met her, she had been working there for only about two weeks. Jerry Nepom was pleased with this new arrangement. "It'll be real nice, because we've worked together a lot in the past, and this will make it much easier. And fun, too."

"How does working with your wife work?"

Nepom smiled. "Why not ask *her?*" He stood up, walked out into the hall and found her. She came in and sat down, a pleasant-looking woman with a nice laugh and eyes that revealed a sharp mind.

"It's not that common to see a husband and wife working together in science or medicine," I remarked.

Barbara Nepom laughed. "Yes, we get a lot of comments like, 'How do you *do* that, twenty-four hours a day together?'"

I said, "Actually, I'm curious about how it works, especially now that you are both in the same lab."

"Well," said Jerry, "I think it actually helps a lot. It's more relaxing and more fun to know what the other is doing. We talk about it all day long, so when we get home, we *don't* have to talk about it. We can devote that energy to our daughter and to family life."

"We really don't carry it home much," Barbara agreed. "If there is something big that one of us is working on, we can just mention it to the other person and at once get a response. There isn't this feeling like you are compartmentalizing your life. A lot of people who are married to folks in totally different fields, they sort of have to 'get away from what I do' and all that. From what I've seen of people in science with partners in other fields, they may say, 'Oh, such-and-so worked out really well.' And their husband or wife may say, 'Uh, what was that again?' and they have to explain everything. And the response to that may be, 'Oh, forget it.'

"Also, things are so hectic right now, that we *don't* always see each other that much during the day. Sometimes we do have to spend more time at home talking about business. Or on the ferry."

"Ferry?"

"We live on Bainbridge Island," explained Barbara. Bainbridge is across Puget Sound from mainland Seattle.

"Which gives us a half hour going and coming to unwind and catch up," added Jerry.

"What's your daughter's name?" I asked. "How old is she?"

Jerry smiled. "She's one and a half years old, and her name is Jessica. Here." He pulled out his wallet. "I just happen to have a picture . . . !"

"Uh-oh! There you are, you said the magic words," said Barbara.

Her husband took the picture out. Jessica Nepom looked like a cute kid. Eating lunch. With food all over her face.

"Do you happen to have a cover illustration for your book yet?" Barbara asked jokingly. Or was she joking? I wasn't sure.

Gerald and Barbara Nepom had first met one another in college, and gotten married in graduate school in 1971. They actually started working together in Boston in 1980. The immediate connection was Mark Green, one of Jerry Nepom's collaborators, who was working in the same laboratory as Barbara. When Jerry made the decision to leave Boston and come to the Pacific Northwest, they both knew it was hard for couples to be recruited together. In their case, though, luck and talent was on their side. Barbara was being recruited for a pediatrics position, and Jerry was being recruited for a medical genetics position, both in Vancouver, B.C. They came to the Northwest for life-style reasons, said Jerry. "It's a lot more relaxing living here.

"So, anyway, on our way to B.C., we stopped in Seattle to visit some friends—and got recruited *here*. We never did complete the Vancouver leg. Barbara hadn't finished her fellowship in Boston completely, so she did her last research year in my lab at the Hutchinson. Then we worked independently. And now we're back together."

"Jerry always wanted to do research," said his wife, "and ended up moving to immunology, with mice and all that. He was not really disease-oriented. But I always knew I wanted to go into pediatrics, and I met a woman who became my adviser, and I ended up doing pediatric rheumatology and arthritis. I went at it from the clinical side, Jerry went into it through straight research. Then he wanted to get more clinically relevant. And we ended up kind of in the same field.

"The nice thing about working together is, you never worry about whether the other partner in the collaboration is doing her or his part of the job. You *know*."

One question, a slightly uncomfortable one, popped into my head. I asked, "Are there ever any jealousy problems with other people in a lab or in a collaboration? Since you're husband and wife?"

Barbara Nepom shook her head. "Not yet. We stay aware of that as a possibility, but it hasn't happened yet. We're pretty careful. But this is the first time where it really could be a problem, because Jerry is the head of the lab, and I'm in an equal position with others below him. But, you know, I have to go and get my own grants like everyone else."

Rheumatoid arthritis, Barbara Nepom's area of research, is an inflammatory form of arthritis. Large growths of tissue form in a person's joints and eat into the cartilage and bone. That decreases the victim's ability to move the affected joints. The affliction is accompanied by pain, swelling, and redness of the affected areas. Rheumatoid arthritis (often abbreviated to RA) most often strikes people in their twenties and thirties. Some people think the immediate cause is a still-unidentified agent (perhaps a virus) that is able to infect people with a genetic weakness for RA. But there is a definite autoimmune component to RA, also. Blood and body fluids of people suffering from RA have high levels of antibodies against the tissues in their joints. Obviously, the body is attacking itself. Whether that is a cause or an effect of RA has been a big puzzle.

That autoimmune connection for rheumatoid arthritis was effectively illustrated in work done by David Yocum of the University of Arizona. Yocum's goal was to find some kind of treatment for people suffering from RA, a treatment that might take advantage of the disease's autoimmune connection. He turned to Cyclosporin A, the drug based on a mushroom found in Switzerland. It is currently the treatment of choice to prevent transplant rejection.

A kidney or heart from another person carries that person's MHC-encoded Self-markers. That person's own immune system, of course, sees those molecular markers and knows that this organ is part of itself. For the person receiving the transplant, however, those MHC markers are nothing more or less than foreign antigens. The immune system mounts an attack against the invading, transplanted tissue. The rejection process involves something called the *mixed lymphocyte response*. This is what happens when T cells from two different people are mixed together. The T cells of each individual respond to the MHC antigens of the other by becoming activated. They go through the stages of differentiation and proliferation, maturing into full-fledged, active T cells. They include killer T cells and several kinds of helper T cells, such as delayed hypersensitivity T cells and amplifying T cells. The amplifying T cells then release interleukin-2, which stimulates the killer Ts into full action. This is almost identical to the way the cellular immune response deals with invading viruses. Cyclosporin A works by suppressing the activity of the T cells involved in the rejection response.

When it was first used in patients receiving organ transplants, Cyclosporin A had results so dramatic that even normally cautious scientists used words like "amazing" and "revolutionary." And the drug is just that. It is also highly toxic, with some serious side effects, including damage to the kidneys and high blood pressure. But it does work, and since the alternative is loss of the transplanted organ—and often death—most patients and their doctors are willing to accept the side effects of Cyclosporin A.

Yocum began his project while he was at the National Institutes of Health. He conducted a two-year study, giving RA patients doses of Cyclosporin A that were small enough to avoid both unpleasant side effects and *severe* suppression of the immune system. The results were impressive. The drug significantly reduced the swelling and pain in the patients' arthritic joints. More than 80 percent of the people in the study also had improved ability to walk and to grip with their hands and fingers. What makes the results even more impressive is that they took place in patients that Yocum has called "the toughest ones"—those whose symptoms have resisted other treatments for rheumatoid arthritis.

Yocum has said that Cyclosporin A "heralds an exciting new class of drugs that are more specific and less toxic to the patient." Other immune-suppressing drugs have been used before Cyclosporin A to treat RA. But they were very nonspecific in their effects, suppressing the entire immune system and thus putting patients at considerable risk of illness from other causes. Cyclosporin A, since it is more specific in its effect on the immune system (suppressing only the activities of helper and killer T cells), may be more effective and have fewer serious side effects than the other drugs.

"We have here a drug that offers these patients a promise of improvement where there seemed to be little hope, and a chance at a better life as a result," Yocum has said.

In fact, the possibilities may be even better than that. Cyclosporin A has actually *cured* rheumatoid arthritis in animal studies. A cure for humans might be possible when scientists can pinpoint the earliest stages of RA in people as they can already in animals.

This powerful immune-suppressing action was interesting to researchers and doctors working with people afflicted with other autoimmune diseases—including Type I diabetes. Early use of such a powerful immune-suppressing drug might be able to stop the destruction of the islet cells of the pancreas. That in turn could lead, at the least, to a slowdown of the process of juvenile-onset diabetes. As 1987 drew to a close, a Canadian researcher reported that Cyclosporin A did indeed have such an effect.

In 1984 John Dupré, a researcher at the University of Western Ontario in London, Ontario, and his coworkers had carried out a small test of Cyclosporin A on people with Type I diabetes. He found that about half of the forty-one people treated were able to stop insulin therapy if given Cyclosporin A. This first study ran for a year, and the results remained consistent.

Dupré's next study was larger, a clinical trial involving 188 people in Canada and Europe. Some of the people had Type I diabetes; others did not, and served as the controls. Part of each group got Cyclosporin A and the rest got a placebo. Dupré's results were dramatic. After one year, 25 percent of the diabetics who had received the Cyclosporin A therapy no longer needed their insulin injections. The insulin-making cells in their pancreases were now producing enough insulin on their own. By comparison, only 10 percent of the Type I diabetes patients who got the placebo had been able to give up their insulin injections. Dupré also found that the earlier the diabetics received Cyclosporin A treatment, the more likely it was that their disease would go into remission. About 30 percent of the people who began the therapy within two weeks of beginning insulin use eventually went into remission, as compared to just 3 percent of the people in the control group.

These results are exciting—but no one should get too excited yet. For one thing, Cyclosporin A is not a cure for Type I diabetes. Dupré found that most of the patients in his first study suffered relapses into active Type I diabetes when the Cyclosporin A therapy stopped. Such therapy would have to continue indefinitely to be effective. Cyclosporin A is a powerful drug, often with very serious side effects, and long-term treatment with it could be devastating.

Such a Hobson's Choice might not be necessary if the onset of Type I diabetes is detected very early. Jerry Nepom's work is beginning to have just such a payoff, a payoff in new commercially available diagnostic tests for Type I diabetes.

Jerry Nepom's work on diabetes was now, in his words, "going gung-ho. We're having some contacts from biotech companies who want to commercialize our work as diagnostic tests."

"Can you mention names of companies who have contacted you?"

Nepom looked at the ceiling. Looked at me. Smiled. "Well, I *can* tell you, but it's probably not something you should mention in the book." He was silent a moment. "I'm trying to think if any of the contacts we've had should be considered to be confidential or not." He shrugged. "I frankly don't know."

"Well . . . can you say where the companies are *located?*"

"Hmmm. One company is in San Diego. There's one in New York, and two local companies, here in the Seattle area.

"The one in New York is actually interested in licensing the technique we developed for spotting the genes that determine whether or not you will have the susceptibility to come down with juvenile diabetes. They want to license that technique and use it to run a reference service. That means they'd collect blood samples from anybody, do the tests at their company, and report the results.

"The other three are interested in licensing our DNA probes and trying to use them in new assays that they are developing. Now, Virginia Mason has no history of doing this kind of thing, commercializing work done here. So what we have done is form a little committee of the Center's board members, and a couple of attorneys who have worked in this general area of industry research and development. The committee is evaluating the offers. We'll probably license the probes to at least one of the companies.

"It'll be kind of fun. My personal style, though, is not to

get too involved in that stuff. I know there are a lot of other scientists who do try to do both—"

"Walter Gilbert," I interjected, "who started the whole genetic engineering revolution." Gilbert, a Nobel Prize winner, had founded Biogen, Inc., one of the first biotech companies. He's now started a new one, Genome, Inc. The company wants to map the entire human genetic code—and then sell parts of it to anyone with the money.

"Yeah," said Nepom, "but, anyway, it's not my style. But I am kind of hoping one of the local companies comes through with the best deal. I'd like to see what happens to it."

While Nepom's diabetes research has attracted considerable commercial interest, the research on rheumatoid arthritis has not. Yet. But there is little doubt it eventually will.

When it does, rheumatoid factors (abbreviated RF) will probably play an important role. Rheumatoid factors are antibodies that attack certain other antibodies as if the latter were foreign invaders of the body. The specific antibodies that become the helpless targets of rheumatoid factors belong to the Immunoglobulin G (or IgG) class of antibodies. Rheumatoid factors were first discovered in patients with rheumatoid arthritis. Later they were found in people with other autoimmune diseases. Most rheumatoid factors are IgM antibodies (which are most often involved with allergies and the allergic reaction), but they can also belong to any of the other three classes of antibodies (called IgA, IgE, and IgG). Researchers know which part of the IgG antibody RFs home in on, and that RF-producing B cells are present in human infants, as well as in adult bone marrow and the bloodstream.

The fact that some RFs are naturally present in the body suggests that they may play a *normal* role in the immune system. Researchers led by Constantin Bona of the Mount Sinai School of Medicine in New York City think there may be two major categories of rheumatoid factors. The first occur in animals (and people) that are disease-prone. These RFs have an inhibitory effect on the immune response, especially on the immunoglobulin G response of the immune system. The second category, Bono and his colleagues suggest, are generated during a normal antibody response to certain kinds of antigens. They're part of that conventional response to an invasion by such antibodies, and so they play a beneficial role in the immune system. For example, they may have a "scavenger role," like macrophages, cleaning up immune complexes (the conglomerations of antibodies and antigens and antigen-studded cells and viruses) from the blood. They might also play a role in the regulation of B cells.

The entire process of susceptibility to juvenile rheumatoid arthritis, and the presence and role of rheumatoid factors, is complex. And fascinating. Barbara and Gerald Nepom had picked a good field to work in, one that had plenty of puzzles to solve.

Barbara Nepom left to go back to her work, and Jerry Nepom took me on a quick tour of the lab. As we walked out of his office, I asked him what he thought the future held for his small laboratory at Virginia Mason? "Well, I think it is likely that the focus of at least part of the lab will shift to the development of gene therapy for Type I diabetes and juvenile rheumatoid arthritis." We walked through a door into one laboratory area. Down the hall to my left, I could see plastic draped over areas under construction. "This is an advantage of a small laboratory. It can stay on the cutting edges because it has a great deal of flexibility," he said.

We walked past benches which had slabs of poly-acrylamide gel sitting around. These were the raw materials of electrophoresis, a standard technique for separating proteins from serum and then identifying different proteins. Each protein was associated with a particular gene. Nepom picked up a transparent piece of plastic which looked like a tiny X-ray negative, and held it up to the fluorescent lights. It was a photonegative of protein blots from one of the gel blocks.

"This is the protein structural identification of polymorphisms. These are two-dimensional gels. Look at this and contrast it with this." Nepom held up a second one. "This line and this line of spots are similar to these lines. OK? These are the markers, the proteins that serve as internal standards. The key spots, the ones we're interested in, run between these two rows. You can see some spots that are kind of similar, but there is one key spot that is there but not—*there*."

I looked. And saw. "Yeah," I said, slightly surprised and pleased that I could see what he saw.

"And this little spot has migrated from *there* to *here*."

"Oh, yeah!" This was kind of fun. I felt a tiny shiver, a thrill. Was this a little like the thrill of discovery? The thrill of new knowledge?

"Now, this isn't a routine doctor's office thing," said Nepom. "It's much more difficult to do this than it is to do a gene probe.

"But look here. This is the key spot," Nepom continued, pointing to a dark fuzzy dot on the negative, "the protein product of the DQ3.2 gene."

"OK."

"This dot, this protein, is the protein molecule that is actually on the lymphocyte cell surface. It's encoded by that gene. If you've got this here, then you have susceptibility to Type I diabetes."

Just inside the door to the lab area, a computer printer was spitting out a graphic.

"This is an attempt to illustrate, in a gene mapping sort of way, the variations that can occur when an individual is tissue-typed for this gene, the DR4 gene. They can have any of these six sets of genes." Nepom pointed to the illustration. "This just illustrates the problem. This, this and *this* gene code for susceptibility for juvenile rheumatoid arthritis. Um, and this, this, and this gene code for susceptibility for Type I diabetes."

He looked up at me. "This solves a lot of problems. When you see it this way, it's simple and makes sense. These genes are very tightly linked. There are only about 21,000 DNA bases between them, and that's not much. They're almost next door to each other. Which is why they tend to go together when you type someone.

"And this is one of our major contributions to the field, that the Type I diabetes gene and the juvenile rheumatoid arthritis gene *are not the same gene at all*. They are linked in some cases, but in some cases they are not linked. We have gene probes to this one here—the Type I diabetes gene—and to this one. So we can now rapidly test for the presence of them."

He smiled. "That's the gist of the story."

5 | Vaccines —
a Refurbished
Weapon

Enzo Paoletti is one of the world leaders in the young and growing technology of genetic engineering of vaccines. His work is revolutionizing the way medical technology will protect people from diseases like the flu, malaria, diarrhea, rabies—and AIDS. Paoletti looks, however, like someone who should have been climbing Mount Rainier. When I first met him, one snowy morning in Albany, New York, he was wearing a checkered flannel shirt, beat-up blue jeans, and what looked like hiking boots. His bushy beard and mustache completed the mountain-climber portrait. He definitely did not look like a sterotypical scientist.

Paoletti's laboratory in the Corning Tower was three floors underground. I got lost looking for it, and finally had to call his office and get an escort from his secretary. As we took several turns back and forth through crowded corridors, my embarrassment at getting lost expressed itself in a feeble attempt at a joke. "Ah, this is sort of like the movie *The Andromeda Strain,*" I said, "where they had the lab deep underground. Hope you're not fooling around with weird alien viruses."

She smiled and shook her head. "I don't think so," she replied.

A *vaccine* is a compound that's designed to do harmlessly what the body itself does after having been ill. A person who has contracted diphtheria, say, or chicken pox, will usually never get that illness again. The immune system's successful defense of the body against the disease has left behind a collection of immunologic memory cells. These lymphocytes are primed to remember the shape of the particular antigens associated with that disease. The next time that virus, bacterium, or toxin enters the body, the immune system's memory cells leap into action. The invader is destroyed before it ever has a chance to begin harming the body.

The whole purpose of a vaccine is to do the same thing, but without the risk of illness. A vaccine essentially "primes" the immune system against a particular disease by exposing the body to a harmless form of what causes the illness. It could be a bacterial or viral antigen, or a chemical piece of that virus or bacteria, or a weakened form of bacterial toxin. The immune system quickly recognizes the antigen as foreign and creates antibodies against it, leaving the body with immunological memory for that antigen. If a virus with an antigen similar to the harmless variant should later invade the body, the immune system will produce antibodies that swiftly attack the virus and destroy it.

There are four general classes of vaccines. First of all, there are vaccines made of living infectious organisms whose virulence has either been weakened or completely removed. The vaccine against smallpox fell into this category. So does the Sabin polio vaccine.

The second category is vaccines made of infectious agents that have been killed. The Salk polio vaccine is probably the most famous of these kinds. Vaccines against rabies, typhoid fever, and whooping cough (also known as pertussis) are also killed vaccines.

Other vaccines are made from toxic chemicals (toxins) released by bacteria. The toxins are either attenuated in some kind of solution, or weakened by chemically modifying them into "toxoids." Toxoids are used in the vaccines against tetanus and diphtheria.

Finally, there is a relatively new category of vaccines, called "subunit" vaccines. These are made using immunogenic pieces of an infectious agent, be it a virus, a bacterium, or a toxin. The vaccine against hepatitis B is one of the first successful subunit vaccines for humans. It uses a piece of the hepatitis B virus's outer protein envelope to induce immunological memory in the vaccinated person.

In the last several years the new medical technology of genetic engineering has revitalized the old medical technology of vaccination. Genetic engineering has really made it possible to move forward with the development of new subunit vaccines. It is also revolutionizing the field of live vaccines. And it is doing so with the help of the "original vaccine"—the vaccinia virus.

No one knows the origin of the vaccinia virus. This may seem surprising, since the virus has been used for nearly two centuries as a smallpox vaccine. But the truth is that no one knows where the virus originated.

Smallpox was a highly contagious and sometimes fatal disease that caused a high fever and successively severe eruptions and pustules on the skin. The disease was caused by a virus known as *variola*. It was spread by contact and through the air. Today, smallpox has been eliminated— the first virus-caused disease to be eradicated from the face of the earth. This was accomplished through an aggressive worldwide campaign of vaccination and treatment against smallpox, spearheaded by the United Nation's World Health Organization. By the beginning of the 1980s, smallpox was gone.

The first step toward the elimination of smallpox—and the development of the medical technology of vaccination—came in 1796, with one of the single most important medical breakthroughs in history. British physician Edward Jenner, the story goes, noticed that people who worked with cattle were less likely to become infected by smallpox than those who did not work with cattle. These were people, he found, who had come down with a disease called cowpox. Jenner took some pus from the sore of a milkmaid suffering from cowpox, and scratched it onto the arm of a young man named James Phipps. Phipps had earlier been exposed to someone else with smallpox. The result of Jenner's daring experiment, to everyone's astonishment and delight, was that young James did not come down with smallpox. The process came to be called vaccination, from the Latin word *vaccinus,* "relating to cows." The stuff used in vaccination to protect someone against a disease was called a vaccine.

That's the commonly told story. The truth, however, is a bit more complicated and vague. First, Edward Jenner did not really "invent" vaccination. What Jenner actually did was rediscover a very simple procedure that many others had used many times before. The technique had been practiced on and off for hundreds of years in China, India, and Persia. In fact, at one point a primitive form of vaccination against smallpox was introduced into Europe and England by an English noblewoman, Lady Mary Wortley Montagu, who had been in Constantinople. However, this technique used smallpox pus to attempt vaccination against the disease. As often as not, the person so treated came down with the full-blown disease and started another epidemic. The practice fell out of favor. It was only when Jenner found a way to use a less-virulent form of the disease that vaccination really became something both useful and safe. So the real importance of Jenner's work is not that he invented vaccination, but that he invented a *safe form* of vaccination.

As for the vaccinia virus itself . . .

Most doctors have believed for years that today's vaccinia virus, which was used as the incredibly successful smallpox vaccine, is a form of the virus that causes cowpox. It is true that many of the first vaccines against smallpox came from people infected from cattle. But recent genetic analysis of the vaccinia virus reveals that it is *not* related to today's cowpox virus.

The matter is further complicated by a common practice of Jenner and other early experimenters. They often used as a vaccine some matter that came from an infection of horses. Jenner called it "grease," but it was actually pus from the pustules of horses suffering from horsepox. Horsepox also infects cows and humans. So some of the cows that Jenner was using in his early work may well have been afflicted with horsepox, not cowpox. And virus from a horse or a cow with horsepox was successfully used to inoculate people against smallpox. Is it possible that today's vaccinia virus is actually related to the horsepox virus?

Possible—but difficult to prove. Horsepox was always a rather rare disease in horses. The last documented outbreak of genuine horsepox happened in 1900. The horsepox virus, it seems, is as extinct as the variola smallpox virus, and has been for nearly a century. Both cowpox and horsepox had natural animal "reservoirs"—they existed normally in populations of animals. In this case the animals were cattle and horses. But since horsepox was so rare in horses, one researcher thinks that this virus actually had another reservoir. Derrick Baxby of the University of

Liverpool has written a book about vaccinia, called *Jenner's Smallpox Vaccine,* published in 1981 by Heinemann in London. Horsepox's true reservoir, Baxby thinks, may have been some small wild mammal. Perhaps the virus was "squirrelpox," or "hedgehogpox." No one really knows for sure, but Baxby sees this as a very good guess.

The vaccinia virus does not have a natural reservoir. Whenever it has been found in humans and other creatures, it always turns out to have been introduced because of a recent vaccination for smallpox. In fact, vaccinia *cannot* exist in the wild. It is too weak and unable to spread beyond the one person or animal in which it may find itself. It is truly a creature of the laboratory, where it is used for vaccine production and genetic research. The variola virus, by the way, had no animal reservoir. It could only live in humans and was only spread from human to human.

So where did vaccinia come from? In 1838 the National Vaccine Establishment in England was claiming that its new vaccine strains came directly from the material used by Jenner thirty-eight years earlier. It is impossible, though, to tell *which* of Jenner's several different mixtures they were using. The vaccinia virus is not related to cowpox. It is too unlike the variola virus, which causes smallpox, to be directly descended from that killer, either. And it is difficult to see how a virus as distinct as vaccinia could have evolved within two hundred years from either cowpox or variola major. Viruses can mutate rapidly into different versions of the same virus. But it would take much longer than two centuries for one virus to evolve into another completely different virus species.

So we can only guess. The most authoritative guess comes from Derrick Baxby, who thinks vaccinia is related to horsepox. But there is no way to be sure, because that virus is now extinct, and no one has any old samples lying around.

Perhaps it doesn't matter all that much. What does matter is this: Vaccinia virus may be ideal for an entirely new kind of vaccine, a vaccine that would protect people against as many as a dozen different diseases at once. Some of the most important work in this radically new field, this marriage of the old and new, is taking place three floors below ground in the Corning Tower in Albany, New York.

Paoletti's office was smaller than that of his secretary, and it looked like it was about to burst at the seams. Books and technical journals overflowed from shelves, tables, and chairs, and were piled on the floor. I balanced my tape recorder on one pile, and we began talking. It was one of the most engrossing discussions I had in my journey through the outer limits of immunology research.

Paoletti began with a synopsis of his own journey. "I did my graduate work at Roswell Park Memorial Institute in Buffalo," he started, "which is one of the foremost cancer research centers. I worked as a technician for a year after I graduated from college, in a virology laboratory. It was run by Bill Munyon. He was studying vaccinia poxviruses. And I very much enjoyed the kind of research in that area. I began my graduate studies a year after that and did my graduate thesis with him.

"During that time Munyon made two very profound observations. The first one was based on previous studies he had done at Baylor, and it was that vaccinia virus had a DNA-dependent RNA polymerase. This was the first description of a synthetic enzyme in a virus. It's a mechanism by which a virus could express its genetic information. It often happens in science that observations are made simultaneously, because there is this growing flavor of what needs to be done. And this same observation was also made by people at Princeton. It was important because it proved that these enzymes did exist in viruses. And Munyon's work provided the intellectual basis for the subsequent discovery by Howard Temin and David Baltimore of the enzyme called reverse transcriptase, which is in retroviruses."

"This was back when?"

"Oh, we're talking about 1967. Which tells you how old I'm getting!" Paoletti laughed.

"And you were working with Munyon at that time?"

"Yeah. I'm credited as a coauthor on that paper, but it's actually his work."

"So Baltimore picks this up—"

"Baltimore and Temin, yeah, and it feeds into the other work."

"That's what Baltimore and Temin got the Nobel for, right?"

"Right. And they cited this work by Munyon as the impetus for their work.

"Now the other observation that Munyon made was also important. It was that you can biochemically transform mammalian cells with genes from viruses. To be specific, he transformed mammalian cells that were lacking an enzyme called thymidine kinase into the thymidine kinase-plus phenotype by means of an inactivated herpes simplex virus. This rudimentary observation has brought about a lot of other breakthroughs.

"I was working on these things, and also working on other studies of poxviruses. I got my graduate degree, and then it was time to go do a postdoc. I really didn't have any specific, set thing to do, you know. So"—Paoletti paused a moment and drank some coffee—"there were two labs I was interested in going to. One was Mike Bishop's lab at the University of California at San Francisco, where they were working on retroviruses. The other was with Bernard Moss at the National Institutes of Health [NIH] who was also working on poxviruses. Well, I applied to both labs, and I was hoping I would get accepted by only one of them, so I wouldn't have to make a decision." He grinned. "I got accepted by both."

I laughed.

"Ah, yeah. And I decided to go to NIH. Because I saw that the poxvirus system was sufficiently complicated and of interest to have a really good scientific involvement over a number of years."

Paoletti ended up spending three years as a staff fellow at Moss's NIH lab. Then, in 1974, he came to the New York State Department of Health, continuing his work on poxviruses. "The poxviruses are such a complex system," he explained, "that you could study it for years and years."

However, working with poxviruses was a bit difficult financially. The reason was pretty straightforward—there really was no serious poxvirus disease anymore. "Smallpox was waning by this time," said Paoletti. "The global eradication of smallpox was a complete success by 1980—and that's a marvelous story, you know." What's more, he continued, poxviruses are cytoplasmic. They reproduce themselves in the cytoplasm of a cell, never entering the cell's nucleus and taking over its DNA. Poxviruses are also very complicated, with more than 200 genes in their DNA code. Finally, poxviruses like vaccinia have no oncogenic potential: They don't cause cancer tumors. Paoletti shrugged. "So, obviously, the attractions for the general scientific community just weren't there in this virus group. And that made it hard to get funding, since money was going to things like oncology. But we kept on working as best we could. We kept chipping away."

For Enzo Paoletti, the big conceptual breakthrough came in 1978. It was precipitated by a serious personal crisis. "I was visiting my family in Buffalo. My father was quite ill at the time," he recalled. He looked up at the ceiling, then at the overflowing bookshelves, losing eye contact with me as he recalled a difficult time. "We got back from the hospital late one evening, and we hadn't had supper. So, you know, ours is a big Italian family, and you sit down and Mom cooks something up. Right? So, anyway, after dinner my brother-in-law and I sat around having some more beer." He glanced at me and smiled, perhaps wondering if I was surprised that scientists drink beer.

"Now, this was at a time that genetic engineering was getting a lot of media play. And he asked me what I thought would be the first fruits of genetic engineering, the first commercial fruits, the first product. And I quickly responded, 'Vaccines.' That began a discussion of several hours as he played devil's advocate, trying to understand what is a vaccine, what constitutes a good vaccine, what its properties are, how genetic engineering would bring these products about and so on.

"A few days later I was driving back to Albany on the New York State Thruway. That's about three hundred miles with not much to do. *And it clicked.* If we could genetically engineer the vaccinia virus—make changes to its genetic code, adding and subtracting from it—we could use it to make a genetically engineered vaccine. That vaccine would have all the ideal properties of a vaccine as I had described it to my brother-in-law a few days earlier. It was immediately clear to me what steps we would have to go through to put the system together. It was also immediately clear to me that none of the technology existed to do it.

"So when I got back here, I began chipping away at *that* block, putting together the various bits of technology to genetically engineer the system. And that's basically how this product developed."

"So it comes from your brother-in-law to a flash of inspiration on the New York Thruway," I said. "That's better than a science fiction story."

Paoletti laughed.

"So," I continued, "what's a *good* vaccine? And why vaccinia virus instead of some other virus?"

Paoletti nodded. "Well, first of all, remember that you can never give skill too much credit, and you should never discount luck. OK? OK.

"We had in hand at that time a considerable amount of knowledge about working with vaccinia. We knew that it worked, and that it was relatively safe. And also highly successful. Its success as a vaccine is demonstrated by the global eradication of smallpox.

"Also, there are properties of the virus as a vaccine that are important to keep in mind.

"A vaccine has to be inexpensive. If you have a wonderful vaccine, but you can't afford it, well, it becomes useless. The classical way in which smallpox vaccine was produced was that people would take a cow and shave and wash it. Then they'd take some seed virus, abrade the cow's skin and let the virus infect the cow over a week to ten days. Then they would take a spoon—I mean a plain old spoon—and scrape the lymph from the cow. Right off the skin. And that lymph was the vaccine. So we're talking about something that was *very* inexpensive, pennies per dose.

"Now, I'm sure we will have better conditions of production with our vaccinia-based vaccines. But the cost is still going to be insignificant.

"Next," Paoletti continued, "the administration of the vaccinia vaccine has great features about it. You don't need expensive equipment. The vaccine was administered by dipping into the vaccine a bifurcated needle that picks up the virus and then jabbing the needle into the skin several times. So you need neither expensive equipment nor highly trained personnel. Vaccinators were easy to instruct and train.

"Another feature of this virus as a vaccine is that it is

stable. It was learned that you could even freeze-dry the virus, so that you could store it on the shelf as a freeze-dried preparation for months without its losing potency. You could ship it to any place on Earth without its losing potency. You didn't need refrigeration. This is important when you consider the status of some places in the world that were having smallpox epidemics. They didn't have any facilities for refrigeration.

"Finally, even though there is a clear consensus that vaccination is the most cost-efficient way of disease prevention ever developed, with the use of any given vaccine there is a benefit-risk ratio. That's the ratio between the benefit received versus the risk of adverse reactions. Granted that there were adverse reactions, certainly the benefit-risk of vaccination against smallpox was a considerably good one."

The result, historically, was the elimination of smallpox from the face of the earth. In 1979 the World Health Organization formally declared smallpox extinct. The variola virus was gone, except for tiny stores of it isolated in a few high-security laboratories in the United States and the Soviet Union. Both countries swear they keep the variola stocks only for research purposes. Some people would prefer that even these tiny amounts of the virus be destroyed.

The vaccinia virus still exists, too. But unlike variola, vaccinia is rarely harmful. More than a century of life inside laboratories has weakened the virus to the point that it is very poorly contagious. In fact, there are only a few cases on record now of vaccinia virus causing illness in people. The largest outbreak of vaccinia virus infection, following the eradication of smallpox, took place in December 1980 and January 1981, in Canada. Four of the six cases involved were the direct result of contact with a

Canadian Army recruit who had received the standard smallpox vaccination. There have been other, even smaller, outbreaks of vaccinia infection. In every case the spread of the virus was limited to people with immediate contact with someone recently vaccinated for smallpox. And the people involved, it turned out, had themselves never had a smallpox vaccination.

One interesting case took place in 1985. A fifteen-year-old girl in LaCrosse, Wisconsin, was taken to a dermatologist for an ulcerated lesion on her lip. She also had several other sores and markings on her arms, an eye infection, and was suffering from a low grade fever and fatigue. Samples of the skin lesions were sent to a laboratory and turned out to have vaccinia virus in them.

The girl's doctor inquired about her medical history. Had she ever been vaccinated for smallpox? It turned out she had, as a child, but had never had the typical reaction to the vaccine. She had no smallpox vaccination scar. The girl was treated with antibiotics and vaccinia immunoglobulin (antibodies to vaccinia virus), and she recovered completely.

The story doesn't end there. The girl, it seems, had a friend who was in the Wisconsin National Guard, and who had gotten a smallpox vaccination at an Army facility at the end of December 1984. The fellow had had a reaction to the vaccination, and the girl had helped ease his discomfort by applying compresses to his skin.

The medical investigation continued. Was it possible that people the girl had come in contact with might have gotten the disease from her? The doctors tracked people down: five family members, and forty-five others who had taken part in a gymnastics competition with the girl in January 1985. However, no one else ever came down with a vaccinia infection.

A more troubling case of vaccinia infection, however,

was reported in 1987. A nineteen-year-old man enlisted in the Army in April 1984. The young man was healthy and athletic, the ideal recruit. He'd had a physical exam before enlistment and had passed. A few days after entering basic training, he got the standard military battery of vaccinations for flu, measles, polio, meningitis, tetanus, and diphtheria. The next week he got the standard smallpox vaccination. For the next two and a half weeks he was fine, and in the thick of basic training.

Then the trouble began. The man came down with fever, neck stiffness, headaches, and night sweats. He was diagnosed as having a disease called cryptococcal meningitis, and the Army shipped him off to Walter Reed Army Medical Center for treatment.

Things got worse. Much worse. Extensive medical tests continued, and they included the diagnostic test for AIDS. It was positive. Confirming tests were, too. The man was neither gay nor a drug user, though he did admit to having quite a few sexual episodes with prostitutes.

Just as significantly, he had never had a smallpox vaccination before the one he received at camp. A month after that vaccination, still at Walter Reed, the man came down with a serious vaccinia infection. The doctors treated him with vaccinia immunoglobulin, and he recovered. But only from the vaccinia infection. The AIDS complications continued, and the man eventually died.

The man's death was tragic, but there was an important lesson to be learned. It had long been known, during the years when smallpox was still widespread, that some people could have serious medical complications from smallpox vaccinations. This was especially true of people with immune systems weakened from a cancerous tumor, or from treatment with certain kinds of drugs. In this case, the man had not yet developed a full-blown case of the illness, but he was nevertheless already infected with the AIDS virus. His immune system was weakened. The injection with vaccinia, instead of protecting him against smallpox, only gave him a serious case of vaccinia infection. His weakened immune system could not fight back.

Perhaps more important, the multiple immunizations may actually have *accelerated* the death of the immune system's T cells. That process had already been started by the AIDS virus (which infects the body's helper T cells and eventually kills them). So the vaccinations the man got against various diseases, including the smallpox vaccination with vaccinia, actually served to hasten his death from AIDS.

And that in turn may be a warning for those who, like Enzo Paoletti, look to vaccinia as a "delivery system" for multiple vaccinations with one injection. Is vaccinia the right delivery system for such a plan in this age of AIDS?

For a vaccine to be effective, Paoletti explained to me, it had to kick-start the immune response. And it had to do that on several different levels. You need a humoral response, a cellular-mediated immune response, and the establishment of good immunological memory. The vaccine has to induce long-lasting immunity. The vaccinia virus, said Paoletti, has all these elements. "It can induce humoral response, and it's also a good T-cell stimulator, which is important. So if one could genetically engineer this virus and use it as a vehicle, you would have many of these benefits," he said.

"Now extend that conception. Look at the classical methods of vaccine production, and you come to understand why a genetically engineered vaccine would be of benefit.

"For example, recognize that if one thinks of live viral vaccines—not killed, but a vaccine à la the Sabin polio vaccine—then the first live viral vaccine was Jenner's. Back in 1796. And the second live viral vaccine was—Sabin's. In the 1950s. There's a large time gap there.

"Historically," Paoletti explained, "there have been two basic methods for making vaccines. First of all, there was the preparation of live vaccines. You isolated the causative agent of the disease, then grew that pathogen in lab conditions that were different from its natural mode. The idea was to alter the properties of the pathogen. That would eliminate the pathogenic properties, but allow the virus to replicate. So this attenuated organism would be used as the vaccine.

"There are significant problems with this method, though. You don't know what manipulations you have to do to attenuate the pathogen the way you want it. And there's always the risk that you haven't weakened it enough. It might revert to its pathogenic state.

"The other classical historical approach," he continued, "was first to cultivate the pathogen in the lab in sufficient quantities. Then you inactivate the pathogen. That process, too, is walking a narrow path. You have to be sure that all the infectious potential of the pathogen is destroyed. Otherwise, you cause the disease. At the same time, you have to be sure that the inactivation process has not rendered useless the immunogenic potential of the preparation. It's a balancing act.

"Now, neither of these two methods is relevant if you can't cultivate the pathogen at all." Paoletti smiled. "Today, for example, we still can't cultivate the hepatitis B virus. Also, neither of these two approaches is useful if you can cultivate the pathogen *but only in small quantities.*

"So. Now along comes recombinant DNA technology. This technology has allowed us to localize specific genes that encode the information for proteins that are antigens, that are important in triggering the immune response. And there are various ways to do that. The idea is, you can isolate that kind of gene from Pathogen X. You splice it into the genome—the genetic code—of the vaccinia virus. Then you can get vaccinia virus to express, or produce, the protein coded for by the foreign gene, which you have taken from the pathogen. You should be able to take this now-engineered vaccine and, in the same way we've always done, inoculate an individual. When you immunize that person, that foreign gene will be expressed as a protein, an antigen. The individual's immune system sees this foreign antigen and is fooled into thinking that it is infected by this entire other pathogen. It will respond to that antigen by making the appropriate immune response. Thus the person becomes immune to that pathogen.

"Now: think back about the descriptions of the historical methods of preparation. In terms of Pathogen X, you do not have to worry about reversion. There is no possibility that you will develop the disease of Pathogen X, because we're only putting in a minuscule amount of the total genetic information.

"Compare that with what happens with an inactivated vaccine formulation. The way the foreign antigen is made by vaccinia is *indistinguishable* from the way that antigen is either made by Pathogen X or the way the antigen is presented to the immune system. Of course, the presentation of the antigen is extremely important in eliciting the proper immunological response."

"It has to have the correct three-dimensional structure which is literally presented to the immune system," I said. "It looks like, say, a cube, and not a pyramid."

"Exactly. Now, suppose the gene from Pathogen X makes a protein normally found or located on the cell infected by Pathogen X. Vaccinia will *also* place that antigen on the membrane of the cell. Not only is the synthesis identical, so is *localization* of that antigen in the cellular environment.

"There's still another consideration here. A live vaccine is a more significant approach than a killed vaccine. The reason is that a live vaccine *actually reproduces*. There's an authentic accumulation of the antigen. The antigenic mass is great, which allows a better and longer-lasting immune response. With a killed vaccine, you usually have to give multiple vaccinations to get you to the level of immunity you'd like. And that approach is not as long-lasting as the live-vaccine approach. A vaccinia recombinant is actually a live vaccine for Pathogen X. It will amplify the antigenic mass and give a much stronger and longer-lasting response."

When most of us think of vaccines, we probably think of polio vaccine, or DTP (diphtheria-tetanus-pertussis), or measles or flu vaccines. In fact, several dozen vaccines are currently available, though not all are considered very effective: two types of orally administered adenovirus vaccine; anthrax vaccine; BCG vaccine; cholera vaccine; the DTP vaccines; a diphtheria-tetanus toxoid vaccine; two kinds of plain diphtheria toxoid vaccine; hepatitis B vaccine; vaccines against influenza; several measles vaccines; the meningococcal polysaccharide vaccine, against various forms of meningococcal meningitis; mumps vaccine (which I wish had been around when I was a kid; it's no fun getting the mumps when you're twenty-three years old); two kinds of vaccine against pertussis, also called whooping cough; a vaccine against the plague; pneumococcal vaccine, to prevent pneumonia and other similar severe illnesses; injected and orally administered versions of polio vaccine; a new version of rabies vaccine; vaccines against rubella and a rubella-mumps mixture; a tetanus-diphtheria vaccine; several straight tetanus toxoid vaccines, a vaccine against typhoid; and a vaccine against yellow fever.

In 1985 a study by a vaccine development committee of the Institute of Medicine in Washington D.C., targeted fourteen disease-causing candidates for accelerated vaccine development in the United States: a new and safer vaccine against *Bordetella pertussis,* the cause of pertussis or whooping cough; *Coccidioides immitis,* which causes valley fever; cytomegalovirus (CMV), a common cause of illness in people with immune systems weakened during organ transplants; *Hemophilus influenzae* type b, a serious illness in very young children; the hepatitis A and hepatitis B viruses; herpes simplex viruses type 1 and 2; *Herpesvirus varicellae,* which causes chicken pox; the A and B influenza viruses; *Neisseria gonorrhoeae,* the cause of gonorrhea; the parainfluenza viruses and respiratory syncytial virus (or RSV), which cause serious illnesses in infants and young children; rotavirus, which causes an acute diarrheal disease; and streptococcus group B, which most often afflicts infants in the first few days of their lives.

After considerable analysis, the vaccine development committee narrowed the list to five primary choices: hepatitis B, RSV, *Hemophilus influenzae,* influenza, and *Herpesvirus varicellae.* Research on vaccines against all of these pathogens continues, and there's been considerable success in the development of new vaccines against hepatitis B and *Hemophilus influenzae.*

"You can use vaccinia as a cassette or a suitcase into which you pack various genes for various applications," said Paoletti.

I said, "Yeah. I've read that the reason we can do these kinds of things with vaccinia is that it is so big. The virus is physically larger so it is easier to manipulate. Is that right?"

"Yes and no. That's a good question. Let's break that down a bit. First, genetic engineering involves the manipulation of *DNA*. OK? We don't yet have the ability to manipulate viruses that are *RNA*. That eliminates using viruses like polio, rubella, and so on. Even if we could, though, there is another drawback.

"Look at the DNA viruses that are available to us. And all the DNA viruses, by the way, have been genetically manipulated. Look at the basic groups. First there's the SV40 viruses, the polyomaviruses. They're very small. They have only about 5,000 base pairs of DNA. So we can only put a small amount of foreign DNA in them.

"Next up the scale are the adenoviruses. They have about 25,000 base pairs of DNA. Again, there's only a limited amount of foreign DNA we can put in. In this case it's because these viruses are encapsulated in a tight, rigid protein structure. A rigid capsule. So there is a limit to the amount of DNA that can actually be put into it without destroying it. Additionally, adenoviruses and the SV40 group have a known oncogenic potential. They can cause cancers. Generally speaking, we probably *don't* want to use such a virus in a vaccine," Paoletti said wryly. "Now, there are adenoviruses that *are* vaccine strains. They can and are being engineered for specific applications. But in general . . . no.

"Now next up the line are the herpesviruses. They're large, about 120,000 base pairs of DNA, and they can accommodate in their more flexible structure much more DNA than the other two groups. The problem, though, is that there is no herpes-based vaccine available. So we don't yet have the knowledge base of a herpesvirus vaccine. Herpesvirus are also known to be able to cause latent infections. That's the basis of recurrent herpes infections. So we'd first have to eliminate their ability to do that. In addition, herpesviruses also have a demonstrated cancer-causing potential.

"Furthermore, if one takes a herpesvirus and inoculates

a person, there is another risk. There are different kinds of herpesviruses circulating in nature. So what can happen is that there is at least the possibility of a combination between what is a vaccine virus and what is circulating in nature."

Paoletti paused a moment. "OK so far?" I nodded. "OK. Now we go up to the poxviruses. The vaccinia virus is a big contrast to these others. It's been used for a vaccine for almost two hundred years, so the medical community is quite versed in its properties as a vaccine. We know that vaccinia replicates in the cytoplasm of a cell, whereas these other viruses replicate in the nucleus of the cell. Therefore, these others have the potential of interacting in an adverse fashion with the cell's DNA. If they don't end up killing the cells, they transform the cells. Vaccinia, which replicates in the cytoplasm, uniformly kills. It is 'lytic,' in other words.

"OK. We know there's a considerable amount of DNA in vaccinia's genome, which is not essential to the virus's viability. We know we can eliminate that without hurting the virus's ability to replicate."

"Ah. So you can take out larger chunks of its DNA without affecting it," I said.

"Right. And we also know that if we don't take any DNA out, vaccinia's genome can *still* accommodate tremendous amounts of DNA on top of what it already has. Whopping amounts. It can easily accommodate two or three *dozen* foreign genes." Two or three dozen additional genes. Vaccinia, it seemed to me, was one hell of a big suitcase.

The matter of extra genes raised a question in my mind. "How do you know that splicing a piece of foreign DNA won't deactivate the virus? Couldn't that happen?"

"Sure," he replied. "And one of the most important things you have to know is where in the genome you can insert the foreign gene without disrupting it, where it's not lethal. You have to find the sites, the loci, where you can do that."

"Fine. The flip side is, could there be a place in the virus's genome where, if you inserted a piece of foreign DNA, you would *make* the virus lethal?"

"Of course. And there is, and was from the very beginning, the question, Are we going to alter the biological properties of the virus by inserting a foreign gene? There is no evidence at all to date that such an alteration has occurred. We as well as others have looked at that very critically." Paoletti leaned back in his chair. "There is no reason to expect, if you think about it, that you *will* alter the virus's tropism to different tissue, or to accelerate its contagiousness. The reason is that the genes which are now expressed by the virus *do not actually become parts of the virus*. The only component of the virus is the DNA, not the *product* of the DNA. OK? The recombinant virus is *identical* to the wild virus in its protein structure.

"That question has been approached from the beginning, and must be dealt with in every new configuration you put together. You do that in a series of steps. You begin by looking at the properties of the recombinant virus in the lab, in tissue cultures. Then from there you move up to small lab animals. Are there any alterations there now? You just move up the scale. We have four or five years of data now, and there is no evidence at all of altered biology. And that agrees with the consensus of biologists.

"I should also mention something else. This is a generic process. That is, you can also consider using this technology for bacterial diseases, or for parasitic diseases. That's important. The five major parasitic diseases, including malaria, affect one quarter of the world's population. So this fact—that this is a generic process that can be used with parasitic diseases as well as viral diseases—is really a tremendous consideration.

"Here's something else interesting about vaccinia. This virus can be used to infect humans and animals. But it is essentially a laboratory virus. It doesn't circulate in nature. That's important. Even though it's *infectious* for you and me, it is of very low *contagiousness*. OK? So one would not expect this engineered virus to be spread as a contagious disease. Also, that means you can take it from the lab and introduce it into a geographical niche, and feel comfortable it will not spread into that niche. It requires an abrasion for the infection to be set up. That's a critical difference between vaccinia and variola, which causes smallpox. That virus was extremely contagious."

One potential vaccine that was not on the list of recommendations of the 1985 Institute of Medicine report was an AIDS vaccine. At the time of the vaccine study, the cause of AIDS had only recently been pinned down to the virus now called HIV. It was already obvious, though, that an AIDS vaccine would be an undertaking so enormous and time-consuming that it simply didn't fit into the scope of the Institute of Medicine report. Since then, however, the AIDS crisis has taken center stage. Several different prototype AIDS vaccines are under development or in preliminary testing.

Another possible vaccine that was not on the list was a new pertussis vaccine. Perhaps it should have, but the criteria used by the vaccine recommendation committee eliminated it from the top five candidates. Nevertheless, *Bordetella pertussis,* the bacterium that causes pertussis, or whooping cough, deserves special mention. The pertussis part of the DTP vaccine is the culprit in the rare cases of severe side effects in children getting DTP vaccinations. Occasionally the side effects have included brain damage, and even death. DTP has become the archetypal case in the argument of risks versus benefits from vaccination. Almost all vaccines have side effects. But the basic argument, from the beginning, has been that society as a whole and the vast majority of the members of society benefit from large-scale inoculation against certain diseases. This societywide benefit of good health outweighs the relatively small risk of damage to a few individuals from the vaccine's possible adverse side effects. When doctors in England and the United States began widespread vaccinations against smallpox in the nineteenth and twentieth centuries, that was the prevailing opinion. And it wasn't just the opinion of the medical profession, or of the companies making the vaccines (there were many at the time, and the quality of the vaccines being made against different diseases ranged from pretty good to downright lethal). It was the overwhelming opinion of the populace at large. Remember: these people, or their grandparents and greatgrandparents, knew the consequences of widespread smallpox. They knew it not intellectually, but from life experience. They *knew* the risks from new, and sometimes not wellproduced vaccines, were worth the benefits for themselves, their children, and their grandchildren.

Today, few people in this country have ever seen a child suffer from whooping cough or polio or diphtheria. Societywide inoculations against those diseases have almost eliminated them from our society. When a child does suffer a bad reaction from a vaccine, that side effect looms unusually large in our consciousness. Perhaps, some say, it's better not to vaccinate our children against these illnesses. No one gets them anyway. . . . But when mandatory pertussis vaccinations were discontinued in parts of England a few years ago, a whooping cough epidemic swept through the population. Some parents learned the hard way that the benefits were worth the risks.

The problem with the pertussis vaccine, unfortunately, has been that it's a crude vaccine. Made from whole killed pertussis bacteria, it has always had a fairly high rate of

side effects. An improved pertussis vaccine is now possible
with genetic engineering techniques. In fact, since the
release of the Institute of Medicine report in 1985, considerable progress has been made on a new pertussis vaccine.
One should be ready shortly.

With so many possible directions in which to move with
genetically engineered vaccines, I asked Paoletti what his
laboratory was now working on.

"We're looking at the vaccinia approach to putting an
AIDS vaccine together," Paoletti replied. "To express
AIDS genes in vaccinia. We have begun with the obvious,
and there is a promise to it. But we have yet to address
some of the questions. We know how to do it in terms of
engineering, but we don't know the significance of the
engineering in terms of protection, of a good vaccine. It's
exciting because it is a unique virological problem."

"But we have a long way to go," I said.

"I think so, yeah. A long way to go."

"How many years down the road? Take a guess."

Paoletti paused for a long moment. "I would say . . .
within five years, maybe sooner. I think it will come about
because it is a serious problem. And it is being addressed in
many places as a serious problem. I mean, forget the
monetary return. That'll come. But it is receiving great
attention from many people. There is just, by the nature of
the problem, the need to test, modify, and retest."

As I got ready to leave that afternoon, Paoletti asked if
I had ever heard of Jean-Pierre Rampal, the world-
renowned flutist. I had. Well, he replied, Rampal was
giving a concert that evening. Paoletti's daughter was a
flutist, and the two of them were going to the concert.
Would I like to join them? He could get an extra ticket. I
accepted his invitation at once. Paoletti gave me his home
phone number, in case something should come up that

would change my plans. As it turned out, something did.

My stomach.

By early that evening I had come down with a bad case of stomach flu. I wasn't so ill that I couldn't appreciate the irony of my situation. Here I was, interviewing one of the world's experts on viruses, vaccinia, and the genetic engineering of new vaccines—and I had been felled by the flu virus going around that winter. I called Paoletti, cancelled our evening get-together, and rescheduled our meeting the following morning to the afternoon.

That night, as I tried to get to sleep, I recalled my flippant comments to Paoletti's secretary about "Andromeda strains" and the lab's subbasement location. It didn't seem all that funny now. Of course, it really was only a stomach flu virus I'd succumbed to, and I was feeling much better by the following afternoon. I ventured out into the snowstorm that had hit the city. A city bus got me to my destination, and I slogged through the wind-driven snow to my next meeting with Paoletti.

Down below ground, ensconced in Paoletti's snowfree but cramped office, I inquired about one of the concerns surrounding the use of vaccinia for genetically engineered vaccines. "In one of your papers," I said, "you talk about 'multiple rounds of revaccination.' Do you mean doing it over and over again?"

Paoletti glanced off to one side, thinking. "Let's say that next year we are ready with a vaccine against hepatitis and herpes, and we put them in the same virus," he began. "And we go out and immunize people against these two. Now, let's say that three years from now we have been able to put an AIDS vaccine together, and a malaria vaccine. The question is now, Can we go back to the same people and vaccinate them against AIDS and malaria; or are we going be restricted from doing so? Because the first time around, *we also immunized these people against vaccinia itself.*"

"Aha. Because vaccinia is the substrate for the other two."

"Exactly! Now, there are a number of parameters. First, when there was an active immunization program against smallpox, the rule of thumb was that people should be revaccinated every three to five years. The reason for that rule of thumb is that the immunity toward vaccinia is not all that high. OK? It falls off significantly after the third year. After about ten years immunity against it is barely detectable, and after twenty years it's almost all gone."

The revaccinations, in other words, acted as booster shots, reactivating the immunization against the disease.

Paoletti paused. "We're not interested in revaccinating people against vaccinia though. We're just using the virus as a vehicle. Granted that three years from now you'll still have some antibodies left against vaccinia. But we know you're not sterile in terms of a potential vaccinia infection. We *will* be able to infect you. But because you have residual immunity, you will bring that infection, that immunization, under control faster than someone who is naive.

"We're interested, though, in immunity against *foreign pathogens.* So all we have to consider is the activation of the *foreign* gene. The way to get around this apparent problem is, you make the foreign gene produce very high amounts of its specific protein. You may have a more restricted replication of vaccinia on subsequent immunizations. *But* the foreign gene's product, the protein it codes for, is made at such high amounts that you will still be well immunized against that new antigen. That's what we demonstrated in that paper in *Science* in 1985."

"How long does it take to go from start to finish?"

"In the lab?"

"Right."

"Hmmm." Paoletti cocked his head and smiled. "Suppose when you came here today you brought us a gene to express in vaccinia. Two weeks from now we would have a vaccinia expressing that gene. Then it would depend on what kind of animal studies to do."

"Suppose I want you to test it in rabbits," I said.

"Weeks."

"Still weeks?"

"Yeah. Maybe four weeks to get enough of the virus."

The technology of genetically engineered vaccines was more developed than I had realized. Still new, yes, but moving quickly toward greater maturity. What was next? I wondered, and asked him.

"How far down the road are you?" I said. "What kinds of things are you working on?"

Paoletti nodded. "Our program now is in three areas. The first area is fundamental research on the vaccinia virus itself. We have been, are now, and will be trying for years to come to understand better the biology of vaccinia. How it functions, the question of adverse reactions to it. How its expression of its genes is regulated. In this area we're making progress. We are doing research on how to regulate the expression of a gene at this level, or that level, or another level. And we're making progress there, too. But it is a very time-consuming effort.

"The second major area of the lab is the development of vaccines. That falls into two areas: veterinary and human.

"On the veterinary side, we are looking at a variety of infectious diseases and developing vaccines directed against them. These are for a variety of species: cats, dogs, cattle, swine, and so on. We have also begun the development of another poxvirus, fowlpox, which can be used as a vector for the poultry industry.

"The program on the human side involves mainly malaria, hepatitis, herpes, AIDS, Burkitt's lymphoma, measles, and a variety of others," said Paoletti. "All of these studies are going on at the same time, and they're at various stages of progression. The vaccines developed on both sides—veterinary and human—are also at various stages of testing. Some are at the first stage, of tests on lab animals. Some are actually at the stage where we expect them to be going into commercial production by"—he paused a moment—"oh, the end of 1988."

"Have you fit more than three genes into a virus and made it work?"

"We have done that, but understand, those studies are done mainly for model-building. Yeah, we've fit in a couple more, but that area is waning, because we are putting the real thing together for real species.

"You see," Paoletti explained, "we had to demonstrate first that the relative location of where you would place these genes within vaccinia did not matter. That the expression of one antigen didn't adversely affect the expression of another. And that the immunological response to one antigen did not dampen or suppress that of another.

"All of that has been demonstrated.

"Now," Enzo Paoletti said, with excitement in his voice, "we are starting to put together the real components of genetically engineered vaccines."

6 AIDS – the Great Invader

The difference between January in Boston and June in Washington, D.C., can be dramatic. The landscape is different, and the weather is different. In January 1987 I was talking with Dr. Richard Thorne at the headquarters of a smallish biotech company named Cambridge Bio-Science, Inc. We talked about, among other things, the deadly disease AIDS, Acquired Immune Deficiency Syndrome. We discussed his company's role in developing a new test to detect the presence of the virus that causes AIDS, and the search for a vaccine to prevent it. The landscape was pure New England; the weather was snowy and cold. Thorne and I were more or less alone during our conversation. My only real problems had been negotiating an icy highway to get to my meeting place, and then doing it again to get back to Boston.

Six months later I was attending the Third International Conference on AIDS at the Washington Hilton Hotel in

150

Washington, D.C. The differences in landscape, weather, and other conditions could not have been more stark. Washington was so hot and humid that walking outside was like walking in a sauna. Several days it rained, making the comparison still more apt. There was no relief to be found inside the hotel. "We expect more than 5,000 scientists and over 500 reporters and technicians," announced the "Memorandum to News Media Planning to Attend AIDS Conference" I had received a month earlier. In fact, more than 6,000 scientists and *1,200* reporters and technicians turned the Washington Hilton into a multistory sardine can. It was almost impossible to move around in some areas of the hotel. The Media Room, at one end of a long, curving corridor, was often a crowded sweatbox. On the first morning of the conference, the city fire marshal walked in, looked around, and told the hotel that the conference *had* to close registrations—period. It was too crowded for safety.

That first morning, I moved from one session to the next, jotting down notes of my first impressions of the crowds, the conditions, and the craziness, as well as gathering tidbits of information about AIDS. The conference was running four to five presentations at once, in different meeting rooms. Every one of the small rooms was packed to capacity. The corridors were jammed. The giant ballroom used for the plenary sessions and major speeches was filled to overflowing. The cavernous Exhibit Hall, with its row of displays by companies, laboratories, universities, governments, nonprofit AIDS organizations, and—in one awful case—a *pro*-AIDS neo-Nazi organization, was not quite as full. But even there it was still easy to catch an elbow in the ribs.

The conference was being blitzed by media attention. It was the single largest gathering of reporters I had ever experienced. I had earlier covered three major interplanetary space probe flybys at the Jet Propulsion Laboratory in California, and had been impressed by the crush of reporters and writers that had swarmed in to cover them. But the 1987 AIDS Conference made the interplanetary flybys look like Girl Scout tea parties. *This* was the Ultimate Media Zoo: one reporter for every five scientists. It was an incredible ratio of notebooks and cameras to brains.

AIDS.
Acquired Immunodeficiency Syndrome.
The New Plague. The Great Invader.
The killer of gay men, hemophiliacs, drug addicts.
Babies.
Women.
"Straight" women.
"Straight" men.
The killer of someone I had known.

How does it happen? A virus known as *HIV* (for Human Immunodeficiency Virus) infects several different cells of the immune system: the helper T cells, some B cells, and some of the macrophages. The virus homes in on a particular molecular receptor that is found on all helper T cells, called the T4 (more commonly now, CD4) receptor. The same receptor is often found on macrophages and some B cells. It has also recently been found to exist on some cells in the brain.

The AIDS virus is different from most. Nearly all living creatures use DNA as their genetic material. DNA is the "master pattern," a template from which the cell makes ribonucleic acid (RNA), which then carries the genetic instructions used to create proteins. This is generally true of viruses as well as other forms of life. However, some viruses exist which use RNA as the genetic material, instead of DNA. These are called *retroviruses*. RNA is the

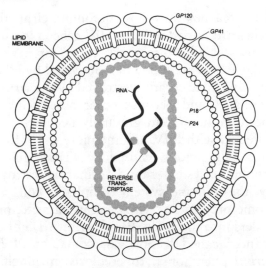

The AIDS virus, HIV-1, is a sphere about four millionths of an inch wide. Its outer membrane of fatty material is studded with glycoproteins gp41 and gp120. Inside the virus is a spherical core of the protein called p18 and a caplet-shaped inner core of the protein p24. At the center is the viral RNA, as well as the reverse transcriptase enzyme that gives the virus its ability to reproduce. *(From "The AIDS Virus," © 1987 by Scientific American Inc. All rights reserved.)*

template to make DNA. The virus then uses an enzyme called reverse transcriptase to insert the DNA copy into the target cell's own genome. The viral DNA lies dormant within the cell. When it becomes active again, it can "hijack" the cell's genetic machinery.

All retroviruses work in this manner, and HIV is a retrovirus—not the first known to infect humans, but the most devastating in its effects.

The helper Ts usually produce chemical factors like interleukin-2, which stimulates the B cells of the cellular immune response to make antibodies against the invading virus. Now, though, the T cells are infected with HIV, which has essentially taken over the T cells' genetic code. The virus uses its reverse transcriptase literally to splice its own genes into those of the T cell.

Then, for reasons only now becoming clear, the AIDS virus's genes are turned on. The HIV gene takes over the T cell and uses it to make more copies of itself. In the process, the T cells are killed or inactivated by HIV. Many B cells are also infected and destroyed by the virus, as well as macrophages and perhaps other nonspecific immune cells. The immune system gradually becomes weakened. People infected with HIV become more likely to contract opportunistic infections, caused by viruses and bacteria that the immune system would ordinarily destroy.

Finally, the immune system completely collapses. Victims become prey to any virus, germ, parasite, or fungus that wanders into the body. People with AIDS often die of a rare cancer called Kaposi's sarcoma, or of *Pneumocystis carinii* pneumonia, tuberculosis, meningitis, parasitic invasions, rampaging fungal infections. In the end, there is little left of the once-whole human being but a wasted, stringy bag of flesh and bones.

And for many people with AIDS, an even worse symptom crops up—dementia. In 1985 researchers first found evidence that HIV was present in the brain tissue and spinal fluid of AIDS patients, directly infecting—and affecting—the nervous system as well as the immune system. Later they discovered why, and how. Many neurons, it turns out, have the same CD4 receptors on their surfaces that helper T cells carry. HIV was plugging into those receptors on neurons, and infecting them. The result was eventual dementia and other mental impairments.

At first it was thought that the effects of HIV on the brain didn't appear until the HIV infection was very advanced, and the victim was near the end of life. It now appears that is not correct. In fact, many neurological effects linked to HIV infection in the brain may begin taking place early on. Researchers at the University of California and Veterans Administration Hospital in San

Diego found that the mental impairment rate in people with full-blown cases of AIDS was 87 percent. In those with ARC (AIDS-Related Complex) it was 54 percent, and for people testing AIDS-positive, 44 percent. How early the effects begin is still not known. Just the anxiety of knowing one is AIDS-positive can cause neurological changes in some people. However, these findings should serve as a warning to doctors who have patients that are antibody-positive for AIDS. Even though they may seem healthy, they may already be starting to suffer neurological problems.

AIDS is a horrible way to die.

We do not know why it happens. The immune system does produce antibodies against HIV. That much is certain. In fact, that's how every AIDS diagnostic test currently works—by detecting the antibodies which the immune system has produced against certain proteins made by the AIDS virus. But the antibodies do not seem to do their job very well, which is homing in on and marking the offending viruses for destruction by macrophages, killer T cells, natural killer cells, and other immune system weapons. The reasons for this antibody failure are still not well-known. In the laboratory scientists have observed AIDS-infected B cells and macrophages clumping together in bizarre "multinucleated cells," which lose their virus-killing ability. That may also be happening in the body, though no one can yet prove it. In people with AIDs the ratio of T4 (CD4) helper T cells to suppressor T cells is almost always out of kilter. Instead of a lot of helper T cells and a few suppressor T cells, AIDS victims have many suppressor Ts and very few helper Ts. HIV attacks and destroys helper T cells, and this presumably causes the reversed ratio of helper to suppressor T cells. It's possible that the relatively huge number of suppressor T cells is actually oversuppressing the immune system's response.

In 1988 a report appeared that seems to shed some light

on why HIV can fool the immune system. Dr. Warner Greene of Duke University found a remarkable similarity between some genes in HIV and the gene that makes interleukin-2 for the immune system. In fact, parts of the two genetic sequences are identical. Apparently, HIV can happily lie dormant in the T cells and never cause trouble until the immune system itself is kicked into action by some infection or foreign viral invasion. The T cells then are activated—and so is the lurking AIDS virus. Its similar genetic sequence takes over the genetic machinery that makes interleukin-2. In a real sense, it uses the T cells to kick-start itself into action. It becomes a T cell-killing machine. And the immune system begins its journey to total collapse.

But why is the immune system itself unable to destroy the invading AIDS virus in the first place? No one is still quite sure why. Later on in the infection, it's because the helper T cells are neutralized by HIV. It seems, however, that the AIDS virus is able to enter and hide in T cells and other bodily cells almost as soon as it invades the body. Another reason for its ability to evade the immune system became clear in 1988. Researchers discovered that HIV is able to infect and hide in the cells in the bone marrow that are the ancestors of the macrophage cells of the immune system. If HIV can hide in these cells, which the immune system is programmed *not* to attack, it may be almost impossible ever to completely eliminate them from someone who is infected with AIDS.

In any case, it is unlikely that any cure or preventive treatment will be possible without knowing in more detail the process of immune system destruction by HIV. For tens of thousands of people, that knowledge will come too late.

It will be much too late for someone I had known.

His name was John Sturgeon. We had finished high school together, and then gone on to the same college for a couple of years. We were never close, but we were friendly acquaintances and classmates. I had liked John, in a sort of distracted and distant way. He was a bit too loud and flamboyant for me then, but he still seemed to be a pretty nice fellow.

The high school was Our Lady Queen of the Angels Preparatory Seminary in San Fernando, California. The college we attended for two years was St. John's Seminary, in Camarillo. We had planned to become Catholic priests. Needless to say, that plan didn't work out. We both left St. John's at the end of our sophomore year. John, I am now pretty sure, left because he was gay. I left because I was straight. That was in 1968. Twenty years later, I was living in Washington State and working as a writer. John had died in 1981. Of AIDS.

I didn't find that out until five years later, in a conversation at lunch with a close friend from those long-ago days. "What's your next book?" Kerry had asked. "Maybe something on immunology," I replied. "AIDS?" he asked. "That would be part of it, sure." "Do you remember John Sturgeon. . . ?"

Writing this book became something more than an interesting project. A few months later my friends Juliana Moon and Peggie Wolfson died of cancer. Those three deaths sealed the personal nature of this book for me.

Massive scientific conferences are not very personal in nature. They tend to be exercises in information overload. To somewhat mitigate these effects, the AIDS Conference organizers supplied those who were registered with a packet of information along with their name badges. The news media folks also received one. It included the standard flyers and maps about Washington (where to eat, sleep, drink, party, relax, see statues, etc.). Also included were two books: one the Final Program for the conference, the other the Abstracts Volume, with summaries of most of the reports to be given in the five days. The Final Program booklet was 5 by 8 inches, and about a quarter of an inch thick. The Abstracts Volume, though, was practically the size of a coffee table book: 8 by 11 inches and over half an inch thick, it weighed more than a pound. Hauling those two around all day long became a dreary project. I was only moderately relieved to note that hundreds of other writers and reporters obviously felt as irritated by it as I.

One item in the packet, though, had the potential to be quite helpful. It was "A Reporter's Reference Card on AIDS Testing." I hoped that all 1,200 news people kept it and read it, for it was a certainty that only a small percentage of those of us with the pale blue News Media badges were science specialists of any kind. Probably more than 90 percent of the news people covering the conference were general assignment writers or reporters who had been given the job of "covering the AIDS Conference" with little more preparation than an hour in the local library— if that.

The reference card on AIDS testing was short and to the point:

GENERAL:
• AIDS—Acquired immune deficiency syndrome—is caused by a virus now called HIV (human immunodeficiency virus).
• All clinical tests licensed for the detection of the virus in blood actually detect antibodies to HIV, not the virus. (Antibodies are proteins produced by the white blood cells [actually one of the types of white blood cells, the B cells] which fight specific types of infection.)

TEST METHODS:
- The most widely used testing procedure is the ELISA, or enzyme-linked immunosorbent assay, method. The ELISA method is suitable for large volume testing.
- ELISA tests for HIV are purposefully oversensitive and produce a number of "false positive" results. False negative results are rare.
- All blood samples that test positive are retested by the ELISA method. Those that test positive again are subjected to a different, more definitive test called the Western Blot.
- A positive Western Blot test is considered the most accurate indication of the presence of AIDS antibodies.

INTERPRETING RESULTS:
- A positive Western Blot test does not mean that a person has AIDS. It means that person has AIDS antibodies.
- Current medical evidence suggests that 20% to 30% of people infected develop diseases associated with AIDS within 5 years of detection. Some estimates double that.
- People who test positive by the Western Blot method are considered to be infectious.
- Antibodies to HIV do not appear in the bloodstream until about 6 to 10 weeks after infection. When no antibodies are present, the ELISA and Western Blot are not effective indicators of potential HIV infection. Antibodies usually appear within 12 weeks of infection. [The evidence now suggests, though, that HIV antibodies may not show up in the bloodstream for six months or even more.]

USES OF TESTS:
- Since March 1985, all donated blood has been tested for HIV antibodies. Blood contaminated with HIV has been practically eliminated from the nation's blood supply. . . .

By the summer of 1988, when the Fourth International AIDS Conference was meeting in Stockholm, Sweden, more than 100,000 cases of full-blown AIDS were reported worldwide. Every country on the face of the planet was reporting (or in some cases, reluctantly admitting) cases of AIDS among its people. More than 60,000 people had contracted AIDS in the United States alone. Nearly 30,000 of them had died since 1981, when the federal government began keeping statistics. That's a fatality rate of 50 percent over a period of seven years. Some researchers estimated that by 1991, the number of AIDS cases in the United States would reach 270,000 with 197,000 deaths.

Some perspective on this: About 58,000 Americans died in the Vietnam War. By 1991 American deaths from AIDS will be more than three times that. It will be more than four times the total combined number of American deaths in the Revolutionary War, War of 1812, Mexican War, and Spanish-American War. The total will be more than three times the number of American deaths in the Korean War (54,000). Ten years would have passed since the first diagnosis of AIDS; the war would have just begun, and the fatalities will continue to mount.

There is still no prospect of a cure for AIDS, nor is there any sign on the horizon of a preventive vaccine being available within the next five to seven years.

Early in 1988 the Centers for Disease Control in Atlanta, Georgia, released a report that painted a wide-canvas picture of AIDS in the United States. At the request of the White House, CDC researchers carried out a review of the hundreds of studies that have measured the rates of infection for HIV in America. The data came from health departments, federal agencies, medical research institutes, and academic departments. The surveys studied often differed in sampling techniques and accuracy, and some certainly had statistical biases. So the picture CDC painted may not have had photographic accuracy. But it was the first to pull together in one place all the information in hundreds of smaller pictures.

Essentially, the CDC picture of HIV infection in the United States confirmed the general outline known or suspected for the last several years. The population groups at greatest risk of being infected by the AIDS virus are (1) homosexual and bisexual men, and (2) needle-sharing drug abusers and their sexual partners—heterosexual or homosexual. The rate of HIV infection for those not in the high risk groups—in what is sometimes misleadingly called the "general population"—remains at a fraction of 1 percent.

The CDC estimated that about 2.5 million American men are exclusively homosexual throughout life, and that another 2.5 million to 7.5 million American males have occasional homosexual encounters. Using data from surveys done in 1986 and 1987, the agency concluded that from 20 to 25 percent of the former group are infected with AIDS. That works out to about 500,000 to 625,000 exclusively homosexual men. The CDC estimated that about 5 percent of bisexual men and men with occasional homosexual encounters harbored the AIDS virus. That's about 125,000 to 375,000 men. So the first major risk group, according to the CDC survey, includes from 625,000 to 1 million American men.

The second major risk group are needle-sharing drug abusers and their sexual partners. This is the most difficult group to reach with educational efforts and the one that gives epidemiologists the most concern. This is the group that would serve as the bridge—the "vector," as the researchers would say—over which the AIDS virus might pour into the general population. AIDS-infected men who are exclusively homosexual in their sexual activity are very unlikely to have intercourse with women and thus pass the virus into the exclusively heterosexual population. The National Institute of Drug Abuse estimates there are 1.1 million intravenous drug abusers in the United States. The

CDC believes as many as 335,000 of them are HIV antibody positive. The rates of infection for needle-using drug abusers run from 5 percent to 60 percent.

A third, smaller, risk group includes the 15,500 people afflicted with hemophilia, which is an inability of the blood to clot. Hemophilia is treatable with clotting factors, which until now have come from donated blood. It's estimated that 9,800 of American hemophiliacs—63 percent—are infected with AIDS. Sadly, blood products for hemophiliacs were not treated and screened for HIV until 1985. Hemophiliacs who received clotting factors before that point are almost all HIV-positive. The number of hemophiliacs getting AIDS from clotting factors has come almost to a stop since 1985, but, girlfriends, boy-friends, spouses, and children of hemophiliacs who already have AIDS continue to be infected.

"General population" is a misleading term. Everyone belongs to the general population—homosexuals and heterosexuals, drug abusers and non-users, hemophiliacs and non-hemophiliacs. The Centers for Disease Control, however, currently uses the term "general population" to refer to those people who are not in one of the known AIDS risk groups. The AIDS infection rate for this segment of the population is by far the most difficult to gauge. Few, if any, large-scale medical surveys have been done to determine how many people in "the general population" have been infected with HIV. A really extensive door-to-door study probably won't be done until at least the middle of 1990. For now, all the CDC can do is rely on the well-studied rate of AIDS infection in military applicants and blood donors. No more than 0.14 percent of the people in these groups, which is probably a reasonable subset of the general population, test positive for the presence of HIV antibodies. That's nearly 360 times less than the lowest infection rate reported for drug abusers. Three other recent surveys of the presence of HIV antibodies in "the general population" include a study of 25,000 Job Corps volunteers, a study of 8,668 patients in four hospitals around the country, and a study of 30,708 newborn infants in Massachusetts. They revealed infection rates no greater than 0.33 percent—one third of one percent.

Overall, the CDC estimates that only 0.021 percent of the 142 million Americans not in the known AIDS high-risk groups—about 30,000 people—are carrying the AIDS virus. The total number of Americans who would test positive for AIDS antibodies (which is *not* the same as actually *having* the disease) adds up to between 945,000 to 1.4 million people.

But these are numbers, and numbers hold little comfort for anyone, at risk or otherwise. There is still no cure or preventative treatment for AIDS. Tens of thousands more people in the United States, and millions more worldwide, will die before the key to AIDS is found and finally fit into the lock. It would be misleading to call Acquired Immune Deficiency Syndrome our century's version of the Black Death. AIDS will certainly not spread with the incredible speed of the plague in the fourteenth century. It could, however, be just as destructive of society, culture, ethics, and mores.

Six months before my humid sojourn in Washington, D.C., I was gingerly driving down an icy Massachusetts turnpike to meet Richard Thorne, at the headquarters of Cambridge BioScience, Inc. The headquarters at that time were not, despite the company's name, located in Cambridge, but just outside the tiny town of Hopkinton, Massachusetts. Hopkinton's only claim to fame is that it's the starting point for the Boston Marathon. The company made its name by developing the first successful vaccine against a retrovirus: the feline leukemia virus, or FeLV, which infects cats. Cambridge BioScience had then gone on to create a new and more accurate AIDS antibody test.

My journey out to Cambridge BioScience was an adventure. I thought I was used to driving in winter snow and ice. I had lived for several years in Spokane, Washington, where winter temperatures of zero Fahrenheit, ten inches of snow on the ground, and black-iced roads were not uncommon. But Boston in winter was terrifying. That morning I picked up a rental car in downtown Boston, and somehow managed to make it onto the turnpike without smashing the car or killing myself. The turnpike itself was a surprise. I hadn't realized "turnpike" meant "toll road," even when it carried an interstate route. I'd grown up in Southern California, where they have freeways. Near the end of my trip out to Hopkinton, I wasn't sure if I would have enough coins for the next tollbooth.

When I got off the turnpike, I took a wrong turn and drove ten miles down an icy local road lined with delightful New England houses. Somehow, though, I made it, and finally found the company offices, and Richard Thorne.

Richard Thorne is a tall man, bearded, soft-spoken, but very sharp. He has a dry sense of humor, and laughs easily. That helped make the interview a good one. Unfortunately, the only room in the building available that morning for us was the library. It also doubled as the coffee break area and as a hallway between two other parts of the building. People came and went as we talked. Doors banged open and shut. People paused to pour themselves a cup of coffee and chat. Later, listening to the tape of our talk, I wondered how either of us managed to make himself understood. But we did. Thorne was eager to discuss their new AIDS test, and I listened carefully and took a lot of notes. What I really wanted to hear about was the company's development of an AIDS vaccine. But as

Thorne talked, I became intrigued by the way the company's work on a virus in cats had led directly to advances in tests for AIDS.

CB's laboratory had begun operation at the end of 1984. The board of directors included Max Essex of Harvard University and William Haseltine of Harvard and the Whitehead Laboratories, both prominent in AIDS research. Essex had been involved with work on FeLV, and Haseltine had a long-standing interest in retroviruses. So the company was tuned in to retroviruses very early. CB's first projects, not surprisingly, were aimed at FeLV: a diagnostic test that would reliably detect the virus's presence in cats, and an effective vaccine against the retrovirus. Both, it eventually turned out, would have a major effect on CB's efforts in the field of AIDS.

Thorne began our meeting by placing a colorful box on the table. It was the company's new diagnostic test for FeLV. The test would determine if a cat's blood showed the presence of a protein from the FeLV virus called p27—the p27 antigen.

"Let me show you what we've got here," he said. He opened a test kit and removed its contents. "This is fairly standard packaging," Thorne said, as he unwrapped the packages. I thought of magicians pulling rabbits out of hats, but this was not magic, just very good science transmogrified into well-crafted medical technology.

Inside the first packet Thorne opened was a rectangular piece of plastic with small holes in it. The holes were about a half-inch wide. This, he explained, was the holder for micro-wells. The micro-wells were in another foil pouch. They were small plastic cups sealed with strips of sticky paper to keep the contents free of contamination. Each kit came with forty-eight wells, so a veterinarian could do four dozen tests. Inside each micro-well was a tiny amount of a monoclonal antibody Thorne called "antibody one."

The kit also included an orange tube, looking a bit like a small toothpaste tube, that contained a second antibody which Thorne referred to as "antibody number two." This was an antibody against p27. Finally, the kit contained tubes of two other chemicals Thorne called substrates.

A veterinarian, Thorne explained, puts a micro-well in the holder, and takes off the strip. The vet would then put a drop of the cat's blood in the well, followed by a couple drops of the second antibody from the orange tube. "This second antibody has an enzyme attached to it," he said. "The idea is that both antibodies capture the antigen. Any FeLV antigen in the specimen from the cat will bridge these two antibodies." In turn, he continued, the second antibody becomes attached to the plastic surface of the well.

The veterinarian then washes the micro-well with water to remove any excess enzyme, and adds a couple drops of the substrate chemicals. If any of the FeLV antigen is present, the substrates turn a blue color in the well. If there is no p27 antigen present, the substrate chemicals stay clear. So the test can be read by eye.

The FeLV diagnostic test is being sold for Cambridge BioScience through Norden Labs. CB makes it, and Nordon sells it through their distribution system. The idea, Thorne explained, is for veterinarians to test cats *before* they are vaccinated. Nordon has had a vaccine against FeLV, which it developed on its own. The idea is not to vaccinate a cat that's already infected. It wouldn't do the cat any good. In fact, noted Thorne, that could lead to problems later on if the cat got sick with FeLV and had been vaccinated. "It leads to lawsuits, I presume," he said.

"Why would one want to sue over a cat with FeLV?" I asked.

Thorne shrugged. "Hey, people who own cats have very strong feelings about them."

CB's development of a diagnostic test for feline leukemia virus has direct consequences for AIDS research. Like HIV, FeLV is a retrovirus, a virus that uses RNA instead of DNA. What's more, it is the best-known and studied of the retroviruses. That research began with a piece of the genetic code for FeLV and used that to create the test. The company was to take the same route for the development of a new and more effective AIDS diagnostic test.

The Cambridge BioScience researchers began by looking at the genome—the total genetic code—of the HIV virus. Genes, remember, are instructions to make proteins. At the time I was talking with Richard Thorne, HIV was known to have at least eight genes. Those genes code for internal proteins, for envelope proteins, and for proteins that regulate the virus's different biological processes. One gene creates the enzyme called reverse transcriptase. This chemical is what makes it possible for a retrovirus to insert its DNA into a cell's DNA. In June 1988, at the Fourth International AIDS Conference in Stockholm, Sweden, Cambridge BioScience cofounder William Haseltine announced the discovery of a ninth HIV gene. This gene, Haseltine said, produces a protein that actually regulates the life cycle of the virus. It could eventually lead to new ways of attacking and killing the AIDS virus, but that's still many years in the future.

Thorne and his colleagues, who were working on their new generation AIDS diagnostic test from 1985 through 1987, were interested in proteins made by other HIV genes. Three of the proteins are called *gp160, gp120,* and *p41.* One of the AIDS genes codes for gp 160, which later breaks apart to form gp 120 and p41. Two other proteins, created by still another AIDS gene, are called *p55* and *p24.*

Thorne explained how these proteins are used in AIDS tests. Suppose you do the test called the Western Blot test. First, you grow some AIDS virus. Then you use standard biochemical techniques to separate all the different proteins that make up HIV. "It turns out," Thorne said, "that the p24 protein accounts for about 30 percent of the protein in the virus. That's a big chunk. The p41 protein accounts for less than 4 percent." Tests like the Western Blot test leave a pattern of bands on the filter paper through which the proteins pass during the test. Each protein has its own particular molecular weight, so they end up stuck on the filter paper at different positions. The patterns on the filter paper are like fingerprints. So when you do a Western Blot, you see a distinctive pattern of bands made by the AIDS proteins.

This is pretty simple in principle, said Thorne. "But it's important to use a test that's sensitive *to the antigen you are looking for*. OK? I think people have gotten into using the Western Blot test without critically thinking about what it is they are doing. They run these gels, get various patterns and intensities, and they automatically assume that if it's strong, there must be a lot of antibody there.

"That may or may not be true. There may be a lot of antibody there, or there may also be a lot of antigen. If there's very little antigen, then you won't see much signal. There's 30 perecent p24 in these proteins, so p24 is a very important antigen in this test, you would think. That attitude is changing, though."

Thorne explained that the new AIDS test was to measure the presence of the AIDS virus by detecting the proteins in the outer envelope. That's not p24, but the proteins gp120 and p41. There's very little p41 in the virus, relatively speaking, and hardly any gp120. The Western Blot test is the standard confirming test for the presence of AIDS antibodies, but it's the wrong test for finding the envelope proteins. A different test, called *radioimmunoprecipitation* or RIPS, works much better. "There are a whole variety of these tests. But the method that works best," and Thorne smiled, "is the one we worked out for FeLV."

Cambridge BioScience began its creation of a new AIDS diagnostic test by snipping out the virus's genetic region that codes for the HIV envelope proteins. Their molecular biologists took various pieces of the proteins and eventually discovered which ones were the most immunoreactive. One particular piece, which included the final third of gp120 and the first third of p41, turned out to be very immunogenic. Then a problem cropped up. When the gene segments were spliced into bacteria, practically no HIV protein could be detected. Though the protein piece was very immunogenic, the bacteria were making very little of it. If the company wanted to use it in its new AIDS test, it would have to find a way to make a lot more of it. After a year and a half of hard work, the CB molecular biologists modified the HIV gene by cutting out some parts of it. Thorne wouldn't say more than that, since the specifics were part of the company's patent application for the test. However, they were in fact able to come up with a modified version of the piece of DNA from the AIDS virus which made enough of the protein fragment in bacteria to be commercially useful.

The company also had another problem to deal with. The envelope proteins they were working with are extremely insoluble. When bacteria produce them via genetic engineering, said Thorne, the proteins are in what's called an inclusion body, which is like a little capsule. They had to find ways to make the protein dissolve in water, so they could run it through various purification methods. "The stuff tends to stick to everything," Thorne explained. "The chemists say the hardest part of working with this protein is that it sticks to itself. Finally, our research director came up with a beautiful technique for handling this." He paused. "Which I can't talk about since it's part of another patent application. But he found out how to make it soluble so it could be purified.

"So: now we have a pure HIV envelope fragment. We call it CBRE-3. What we did with it was put it into an ELISA test. You put this recombinant antigen in these little wells, and then you add your serum from the person. If it contains HIV antibody, it will react to the antigen. You wash away any unbound materials and eventually see a blue color that changes to yellow when you stop the reaction. In this case you identify it by eye, so you don't stop it. You let it stay blue." *Voilà!* Detection of AIDS antibodies.

"Current diagnostics get lots of false positives," I noted.

"Yes. And part of the reason for that is that retroviruses, when they're budding out from infected cells, pick up cell material. It's an intrinsic part of the virus. It's possible to purify out those contaminants, but then your yields drop so dramatically that it becomes economically unfeasible.

"Genetic Systems in Seattle did a nice thing to reduce the problem," Thorne said. "They used a cell line that doesn't have certain antigens that cause false positives. There are still other materials there, though. There are nonspecific reactions, which happen in this kind of assay. The antibody sometimes sticks nonspecifically to the antigen, for example. And much of what goes into making a more accurate antibody test has to do with how we manufacture the antibodies—wash conditions, the temperature at which we make the mixtures, how long they're incubated, and so on."

Thorne leaned back in his chair. The room was quiet for the moment; people were finished with their coffee break. "You know," he said, "the number of variables in getting this kind of process right is just amazing. At one point I was working on a bovine leukemia virus test, which is another retrovirus similar to this one. I tried to break the process down into the number of steps it normally takes, and then figured in a reasonable number of variables at each step. I calculated that if I tried to do all those combinations, I couldn't get them all done in my lifetime." He laughed. "It was literally billions of combinations. So there's a lot of room for working these things out empirically."

"Guessing, in other words."

Thorne smiled. Guessing or not, he felt that Cambridge BioScience had an AIDS antibody test that was extremely good and extremely accurate. "I think it has better sensitivity than some of the other tests. The U.S. Army is testing everyone for AIDS, OK? Well, at one point they had over 150,000 people tested, and they found 2,707 positives. That's using the current test. Those positives were then tested with the Western Blot test, to confirm or deny them. About 700 of them were positive in the Western Blot; they agreed with the original test. And about 2,000 were negative with Western Blot. Those are your false positives from the standard HIV antibody test.

"These same 2,700 samples that originally tested positive were also run through our new test, with our recombinant antigen. And it agreed with all but nine. Our test said that nine of these were positive. The Western Blot said they were not. The new test we are developing showed that the nine samples did have either gp160 or gp120.

"So. The Western Blot test said there weren't any AIDS antibodies. Our test said there were, and the standard ELISA tests said there were. We think that indicates that our test is even more sensitive to envelope antibodies than the Western Blot. Since our test would have picked out most of the 1,900 or so true positives, which the other tests did, our test could be used to confirm or deny any antibody-positive results from the first round of ELISA-type tests. And if we get it licensed and through enough testing, it would even be good for the initial antibody screening."

"How many samples have you run through your antibody test?" I asked.

"Our total experience with this is with between 3,000 and 5,000 samples, so far," Thorne replied. "Anyone with gp120 or gp160 antibody has always been detected. The specificity of our test seems to be greater than current tests by a wide margin. But," he added, "I want to be absolutely as critical as I can. The fact is, earlier versions of the current licensed AIDS antibody tests were 'dirty' compared to later versions. Their specificity is increasing. And I think their sensitivity is increasing, too." Then he grinned. "But all that means is they're becoming more like our test. We are certain that we've found the best antigenic sites of the AIDS envelope antibody."

"OK. Right now there are several AIDS antibody tests on the market," I said. "Some are based on Gallo's AIDS virus, and some, like the Genetic Systems test you mentioned, are connected to Luc Montagnier and his people at Institut Pasteur. Based on what you know now, can you tell which of these two kinds of test is the more accurate?"

Thorne shook his head. "It doesn't matter whether it's Gallo's virus or Montagnier's virus. They are practically identical. The Genetic Systems cell line is a better one, but I gather that new test being put out by Abbott, which is based on Gallo's cell line, is also very good. They have cleaned it up.

"So I think that the newest versions of these tests are very accurate, as far as I've heard."

"How much longer before the Cambridge BioScience test becomes a reality?"

"Well, as of right now we're writing an IND application. That's 'investigatory new drug.' Because this is a recombinant material, we have to file an investigatory new drug application. So there's a whole other round of testing we have to do before it goes commercial. The IND application is really a kind of clinical trial. Then we do product licensing. . . ." He shrugged. "I'm surprised sometimes that anything ever gets out onto the marketplace, to tell you the truth. In answer to your question, though, we are shooting for the end of 1987. It's a hectic pace."

"I gather Jeremy Rifkin hasn't found out about you yet."

Thorne laughed. "No."

"Thank God."

He smiled slightly. "We hope that we are actually making the world safer. Even though the current test kit for AIDS antibodies is safe, the people who are making it are certainly at some risk. The risk from the recombinant material we are using, the genetically engineered gp12 protein, is far less. Also, it's much more economical."

"And after this? Is there a third generation AIDS test?"

"Actually," said Thorne, "there's a second and a half generation test." And he dropped a bombshell on me. "What we want to do is use the same antigen on latex beads. That way we can use the test in Africa."

Africa, where AIDS may well have first begun. In Africa AIDS is not a disease that overwhelmingly strikes homosexuals, hemophiliacs, and drug addicts; there, it is well-established and spreading rapidly in the general population, killing tens of thousands, if not hundreds of thousands of men and women. Researchers at the 1988 AIDS Conference in Stockholm warned that the population in some African countries would soon begin to *drop*— because of AIDS. A simple and effective AIDS antibody test would have an enormous impact in Africa.

The new AIDS test Thorne was talking about would work in five minutes. No complex equipment would be needed. In fact, no equipment at all would be necessary for this test. It was so simple to carry out and understand, said Thorne, that anyone would be able to learn to read it. In this way it was like the smallpox vaccine. And its impact coud be just as revolutionary.

"We've tested this one very rigorously already," said Thorne. "Now we're trying to figure out how to get it licensed. We went to the FDA, and they weren't sure, either. They want to help us to get it approved as fast as possible. So we're working on the final product development of this version of the test, and we are very excited about that. We want to get it to places like Africa where they need it. And they *really* need it," said Thorne, his voice beginning to rise with emotion.

In April 1987 CB's IND application for the first AIDS diagnostic test, the so-called RIPS test using gp120, was approved by the U.S. Food and Drug Administration. They could begin human clinical trials of the second generation diagnostic test for AIDS. The company announced they expected to release the test to worldwide markets by early 1988. At the same time, the company publicly announced its intent to file an IND application on the five-minute AIDS test. They hoped they could begin selling this one too in 1988.

Those hopes indeed flowered into reality in 1988. It was to be Cambridge BioScience's breakthrough year. First, in February the company got the rights to an historic patent issued to Harvard University. Harvard researchers led by William Haseltine had found ways to make large amounts of the gp120 AIDS protein using genetic engineering techniques. The U.S. Patent Office essentially ruled that this gave Harvard the right to patent recombinant gp120, and the right to money made from any tests that used it. Haseltine was a cofounder of Cambridge BioScience, and CB got the rights to the patent. Gp120 is the essential protein in the new AIDS test made by CB.

In April, the company applied to the Food and Drug Administration for permission to begin selling the emergency five-minute AIDS test in the United States. And in May, the government gave Cambridge BioScience approval to begin selling the five-minute AIDS diagnostic test overseas to selected areas. Such as Africa.

There was still another factor that Cambridge BioScience would have to deal with at some point. For that matter, the entire medical and drug industry community would have to come to terms with it. If someone—CB or some other company—were at last to develop an effective AIDS *vaccine*, how would doctors diagnose people with AIDS? The same AIDS proteins would be involved in both an AIDS vaccine and AIDS diagnostic tests. A person vaccinated against AIDS, in other words, would test positive for the presence of HIV, even though the virus was not present. Cambridge BioScience, said Thorne, was already working on a third generation AIDS diagnostic test that would get around that problem.

How? "We have to find some antigens that are not necessary for vaccine but which we can use for AIDS diagnostics," said Thorne. "That's about all we understand at this point. Also, we're looking at ways to clone and express the various structural antigens from HIV, and maybe put them in separate wells in a diagnostic kit. That way clinicians could look at what happens to antibody titers in people who are infected. No one can do that, yet.

"Let me say this. It is amazing how much has been learned about this virus in such a short time.

"But," Thorne added, "there are also a lot of things about AIDS that are still unknown."

Six months later, I was pondering Thorne's words as I shoved my way through sweaty crowds of scientists and reporters in the lower levels of the Washington Hilton

Hotel. By the end of the first day, I knew I could never cover the conference with any semblance of completeness. The entire enterprise was simply overwhelming. I had gone through the Conference Final Program, and marked the talks I absolutely had to attend each day. I found there were even too many of those, often with several scheduled at the same time. Not even science writers can be in more than one place at the same time. I found that out the hard way. One afternoon, near the end of the conference, I simply went back to my motel room and went to sleep for nearly fifteen hours. I was completely exhausted.

The conference was by no means a waste of my time, though. It was an exhilarating experience, and the source of new knowledge. One of the most interesting aspects of the conference for me was the discovery of the existence of a whole array of drugs for the treatment of AIDS victims. They may not be cures, but they help. The first successful drug treatment for AIDS patients was with a compound called AZT or zidovudine. Reports at the 1987 Conference showed that it was turning out to be very successful. The great majority of AIDS patients being treated with zidovudine were living much longer. Nor was zidovudine the only hope. Several other drug treatments were in clinical trials. Hoffmann-La Roche was testing a compound called DDC in combination with zidovudine. It's only side effects were sore feet. A drug called Ribavarin was also being tested. Some studies indicated that Ribavarin delayed people with ARC, AIDS-Related Complex, from progressing to full-blown AIDS. Imreg-1 is a drug that stimulates the production of interleukin-2, gamma-interferon, and other immune system regulators. In tests of people with ARC, Imreg-1 seems to improve the functioning of the immune system and slows the rate at which AIDS progresses.

Still another possible AIDS treatment, and one that remains quite controversial, was uncovered by researchers led by Candice Pert at the National Institutes of Mental Health (NIMH). In 1975 Pert was a codiscoverer of the chemical receptor for endorphins, the body's natural pain-killers. Pert and her coworkers have now discovered a peptide (a small protein) which she has dubbed Peptide T. The compound bears a remarkable resemblance to part of the CD4 receptor molecule. One of Pert's collaborators, Swedish researcher Lennart Nillson, injected a small number of Swedish AIDS patients with a preparation of Peptide T. The patients appeared to have a partial remission of their symptoms. Pert thinks that Peptide T could thus be a possible treatment for AIDS sufferers.

Pert's suggestion has met with considerable disagreement—even scorn—from other AIDS researchers. However, Pert is continuing her research into Peptide T. Research in 1987 and 1988 continued to suggest that there may well be something to Peptide T as a medical treatment for AIDS sufferers. It may decoy the AIDS virus away from helper T cells. Peninsula Laboratories near San Francisco is pressing forward with tests of Peptide T on AIDS patients. Meanwhile, reports in mid-1988 from Pert's group were encouraging—and intriguing. Peptide T's structure greatly resembles that of a brain chemical called VIP. By mimicking the action of VIP in the brain, Peptide T may act to protect people with AIDS from the dementia caused when the AIDS virus plugs into the CD4 receptors on some brain cells.

A similar route to blocking AIDS infection was reported early in 1988 by researchers for several drug companies, including Smith Kline & French, Biogen, and Genentech, and people at Harvard Medical School and the Basel Institute of Immunology in Switzerland. These researchers have used genetic engineering to make large amounts of the CD4 molecule, the receptor on helper T cells. They added the excess CD4 molecules to test tubes with helper T cells, then introduced HIV into the mixture. The extra CD4 molecules seemed to trick the virus-to-cell binding system. They adsorbed the AIDS viruses before they could attack the T cells. Even more encouraging was the fact that the CD4 molecules can inhibit many different strains of HIV.

Despite the frustration and exhaustion, I eventually came away from the Third International Conference on AIDS with a sense of optimism. Yes, the federal government was still not spending enough money on AIDS research. Yes, the politicians were still playing politics with people's lives and indulging their private biases. (Vice President Bush, upon being booed by thousands of scientists, turned to someone and said: "Is there some gay rights group out there?"—and it boomed over the microphones and through every meeting room in the hotel.) Yes, there was still an enormous amount of work to be done. There were still many years of death and despair ahead.

But progress was being made, enormous progress. The HIV genome was understood better than ever before; the virus's effects on the immune system were coming into clearer focus. Scores of research teams around the world were designing and testing new drugs to treat people with AIDS and alleviate their symptoms.

And there were the tantalizing reports of new candidate vaccines—the ultimate weapon against AIDS. The counterattack.

7 AIDS – the Counterattack

It was a cold day in San Francisco. The sky was leaden. I had come to the City by the Bay to meet with Donald Francis of the Centers for Disease Control. He was currently "on loan" to the California State Department of Health. Don Francis is the acknowledged expert in the United States on the hunt for a vaccine against AIDS.

Outside the Federal Building, where Francis's office was located, tents and tables were set up on the concrete patio. An AIDS Camp-In was protesting the federal government's low level of funding for AIDS research. Some of the men in the tents and at the tables were suffering from the grim disease. Others "merely" had ARC, AIDS-Related Complex. Still others were friends or lovers of AIDS victims. The wind blew cold along the patio, and people scrambled to keep the pamphlets from fluttering away.

Much, much later, long after my visit to San Francisco, the surgeon general of the United States would remark to

179

reporters that AIDS research would not truly become a national priority until every person knew someone who had died of it. And that day, he warned, was not far off. For me that day had arrived a year earlier. And now, out on the streets of San Francisco, I spent time talking with men for whom that time had also arrived.

In 1986 the National Academy of Sciences declared: "The only hope for halting the spread of [AIDS] completely is widespread immunization."

Somewhere between 5 and 10 million people worldwide are now infected by the AIDS virus. The search is on for an AIDS vaccine, but it will take a long time. It may even be impossible. Researchers at the Third International AIDS Conference, held in 1987, seemed confident that an AIDS vaccine would eventually be found. A year later, in Stockholm, the same scientists were much less optimistic. A year's worth of research and experiments had produced more questions and few positive results.

The problem is that HIV is like no other virus for which human vaccines have been developed. The obstacles facing researchers are difficult—and perhaps impossible—to overcome. Like the influenza virus (to which it is *not* related) HIV can mutate itself into many different variants. That in itself could make an effective vaccine difficult to create. Most flu vaccines are good only against one of a few flu virus variants. When the virus mutates into a new version, the old vaccines become useless. The same thing could happen with AIDS vaccines effective against only a few HIV variants.

It's clear that humans who contract AIDS never make enough antibodies to defeat the virus. What isn't yet clear is whether or not an AIDS vaccine can boost the human immune system into doing what it apparently cannot do naturally. Some victims of other diseases for which vaccines have been made have always recovered from their illness. That includes hepatitis B. This illness is most prevalent in gay men, and the vaccine against it was the first subunit vaccine ever made. Scientists were able to find the antibodies against hepatitis B by examining the blood of people who recovered from the illness. About 90 percent of all people infected with hepatitis B will eventually recover. However, very few people who develop full-blown AIDS (called "frank AIDS" by researchers) survive more than eighteen to twenty-four months. And no one knows for sure yet what the protective antibodies against HIV actually are.

Don Francis is looking for answers to the questions.

In his tiny cubbyhole of an office, Francis leaned back in his chair and talked of the search for a vaccine against this killer. Francis looked a little like the singer John Denver. His voice was calm and clear, but didn't hide his enormous energy and enthusiasm for his vocation, the search for an AIDS vaccine.

The efforts for pursuing a vaccine for AIDS, Francis explained, were (and still are) highly technical. Most researchers, however, have been following an approach outlined in an article written by Francis in the *New England Journal of Medicine*. It was really a standard approach, he said. To get an antibody that protects against future infections, one has to use some antigen to induce that antibody in the individual before the person is actually exposed to the disease. Then, when that person is exposed, the individual will be able to mount a rapid immune response and kill the virus which induced it. That's what's called immunological memory.

"Protective antibodies against viruses have by and large been directed toward the outer antigens of a virus," Francis explained. "That's logical, since they're sitting there on the outside of the virus. You stick an antibody on it, and those antibodies either kill the virus directly or with the help of the parts of the immune system called complement. So, that leads to the death of that virus. It may also lead to the death of the cell which is expressing that virus." That happens because the virus has infected the cell and is using the cell to manufacture more of itself. The virus's surface is budding out of the cell and exposed to the immune system.

Francis continued: "We knew very early on that the outside of the virus is a sugar protein called a glycoprotein." I nodded. "You know what I'm talking about, I gather," he said. Francis was referring to the gp120 and gp160 AIDS proteins Richard Thorne had discussed, as well as another one called gp110. Other HIV proteins, Francis added, lie deeper in the virus, and they include p17 and p41. The immune system "sees" gp120 and gp160, the envelope proteins, first. Only later do the inner core proteins become visible.

The first step of Francis's strategy for finding an AIDS vaccine reminded me of a joke my Budapest-born mother had told me. "The recipe for Hungarian rabbit stew begins: First, you steal a rabbit." Francis's first step was to get some HIV protein, by whatever means possible. Then, in increasingly expensive, increasingly difficult model systems, researchers would see if the protein being used actually induced immunity. "You start with small animals first," said Francis, "then move on to chimpanzees and then finally to humans. Chimpanzees are the only animal we know of outside of humans that are susceptible to HIV itself. Each one of these steps would be 'gated' to success. That is, you take a small animal, and stick it with the protein and adjuvant." An *adjuvant* is a chemical mixed with a vaccine to help boost its ability to prime the immune system. "If that animal makes 'neutralizing antibodies'—that is, antibody that will kill the virus in a laboratory test called neutralization—well, that's one gate you have passed through.

"Then you move on to a chimpanzee. You inoculate the chimp, and if *it* makes antibody, then you challenge it." To "challenge" an animal in immunology is to inoculate it with the actual virus, and see if the vaccine has actually primed the animal's immune system to protect it. "Now, if *that* works," he continued, "if the chimp makes neutralizing antibodies to the AIDS virus, then you move on to humans."

One big bottleneck in the process, however, are the chimps. "We really don't have the system perfected yet" for using chimpanzees in AIDS vaccine tests, Francis said. For one thing, the primates are terribly expensive. It costs about $15,000 a year to feed and house a chimp. Francis contended that there are enough chimps for AIDS vaccine tests, but others have disagreed. The situation is complicated by the current ban on importation of chimpanzees from Africa. What's more, chimpanzees may not be a perfect model for human infection by AIDS. Some chimps injected with HIV develop temporarily enlarged lymph nodes—a sign that their immune systems are responding to the virus—but they do not actually appear to come down with the disease.

Nevertheless, many researchers think that chimps can at least be used to test the safety of prototype AIDS vaccines. Perhaps even the quality of the immune response could be tested in chimps—whether a vaccine induces the production of neutralizing antibodies to HIV, for example. The real question to be answered, of course, is whether or not a vaccine protects the chimps against AIDS infection when they are challenged by the virus. In early 1987, when I first met Francis, no proof of such protection had emerged. Some chimps have shown signs of increased levels of AIDS antibodies. By the middle of 1988, the situation had not changed too much. A test in chimpanzees of a vaccine against Simian Immunodeficiency Virus had been modestly successful. Two chimps had been protected for many months against SIV. On the other hand, Oncogen in Seattle had tested its prototype AIDS vaccine on chimpanzees. The vaccine completely failed to protect the animals against HIV infection.

Another problem with chimps is perhaps just as serious. Simply stated, chimpanzees are in short supply. The CDC's Patricia Fultz may have found an answer to that problem. She has found that some rhesus macaques can be infected with a version of the AIDS virus called HIV-2. Humans infected with HIV-2 have been identified in Africa and the United States. There is still some uncertainty about whether monkeys injected with HIV-2 will actually develop the disease. Even if they do not, though, they could still be valuable to AIDS research. They're much less expensive than chimpanzees, and there are about a hundred times more rhesus macaques available for research than chimps.

Because of the shortage of chimpanzees, and the difficulty of using them for AIDS vaccine tests, some AIDS researchers think it's necessary to move quickly to limited human tests. In fact, Oncogen began testing its AIDS vaccine on a small number of people, even though it failed in chimps. Other scientists, though, advocate moving to human trials of an AIDS vaccine only after animal tests have been used to the fullest extent possible. This might alarm groups who are at high risk from AIDS. Extensive animal tests before human trials would mean many more years before an AIDS vaccine reaches the public. Tens of thousands, perhaps hundreds of thousands, more people will die of the disease. However, extensive animal tests may be the only prudent thing to do. Other vaccines have "gone public" before, and turned out to be inadequately tested. In a case that involved cats, an early vaccine against feline leukemia virus, developed and marketed in the early 1970s, actually *suppressed* the animals' immune systems. Cats who got the vaccine *died* of FeLV instead of being protected from it. (In contrast, the Cambridge BioScience vaccine worked.) Another example involved humans and two measles vaccines introduced in the 1960s. People who received one of these vaccines later became very ill when they were actually exposed to the measles virus, or received injections of some other live-virus vaccine. The measles vaccines had apparently induced improper or incomplete immune responses. The result was damage to the immune system rather than immune protection.

Such a scenario for an AIDS vaccine would be worse than a disaster. It could end up being a global catastrophe.

AIDS is already generating global concern, and one reason is that it still remains poorly understood. One of the biggest mysteries about AIDS is the most fundamental: Why do some people infected with HIV go years without developing the illness, while others succumb within months? Between 1 and 1.5 million Americans are infected by HIV. Statistics indicate that 20 to 30 percent of them will develop full-blown AIDS within five years of being infected. Many researchers think that additional factors, or "cofactors," are the trigger for the actual development of AIDS. The two most common theories center on genetic predisposition, and the action of other viruses or bacteria. If the coinfection hypothesis is correct, then avoiding the second virus could be a key to health. If the genetic predisposition hypothesis is right, avoiding infection could be a lot harder.

The genetic tendency hypothesis is based on the fact that people with frank AIDS have extremely *small* amounts of HIV in their bloodstream. Only one in 10,000 to 100,000 lymphocytes show evidence of HIV infection in people with frank AIDS. Where are all the viruses? One answer is that only a few are needed to cause the syndrome. HIV infection by a few viruses triggers the body's immune system to attack not only the virus, but also the body's own cells. AIDS is the result of an autoimmune reaction, according to this hypothesis. The immune system's different components normally work together to destroy invading viruses without attacking the body's own cells. In the case of AIDS, that process is short-circuited.

First, HIV attacks the all-important helper T cell. The virus plugs into the receptor—a molecular keyhole on the T cell—called the CD4 receptor. Helper T cells ordinarily use this receptor to connect to other immune system cells as part of the normal immune response. HIV may be able to plug into the CD4 receptor because part of the virus's surface "looks" like the parts of other, normal immune system cells. If this is actually correct, then HIV destroys the immune system by mimicking it.

Next, the immune system finally recognizes HIV as an invader. The B cells make antibodies against the AIDS virus. But those antibodies also end up attacking *other* immune system cells carrying the CD4 receptor because HIV resembles them. The antibodies prevent helper T cells from communicating with these other immune cells and short-circuit the immune response. At the same time, the HIV-prompted antibodies trigger the release of a second set of antibodies, anti-antibodies against both the first antibodies and the CD4 receptors on helper T cells. The result: a handful of HIV causes the immune system to self-destruct.

If this scenario is correct—and all evidence at this point is that this is the basic way the AIDS virus infects the immune system—the question still remains: Why do some people come down with AIDS quickly, and others do not?

The answer may be in the differences in people's genetic code. The proteins on the surfaces of immune system cells to which helper Ts attach (via the CD4 receptor) differ from person to person. They are encoded by the person's genetic code, and the coding is inherited. People who have cell surface proteins that resemble the surface of HIV are at risk of suffering an autoimmune reaction to HIV infection. Those who have cell surface proteins that are different from HIV are less likely to develop AIDS.

While some scientists like the genetic theory, others favor the coinfection hypothesis. Scientists at the National Institute of Allergies and Infectious Diseases (NIAID) have found considerable evidence for it. A piece of HIV genetic material was spliced to bacterial genes that produce an easy-to-identify enzyme. When the combination was exposed to different kinds of viruses, they made more of the enzyme. That showed that the HIV gene was multiplying under the influence of the viruses. Later, the researchers carried out experiments using the entire AIDS virus. The results confirmed the first tests. The viruses were quite different from one another, so it is unlikely they were all making the same protein to stimulate the AIDS virus. Rather, it would seem the coinfectious viruses induce HIV-infected cells to produce an AIDS-stimulating protein. In a sense, the infected cell is tricked into killing itself.

Jay Levy of the University of California at San Francisco, one of the early discoverers of the AIDS virus, has found that some people have white blood cells that produce a protein that suppresses HIV activity. This could be a protein that counters coinfectious activity. Other evidence shows a very high percentage of AIDS in people who are also infected with hepatitis B, and with venereal diseases such as herpesvirus, syphilis, and gonorrhea. At the 1988 International AIDS Conference, AIDS virus codiscoverer Robert Gallo announced additional proof that the presence of the hepatitis B virus made people much more likely to come down with AIDS.

The two theories—coinfection and genetic predisposition—are not mutually exclusive. Each could be the operative mechanism in different people. But which is correct—if not both—is still an open question. The eventual success of an AIDS vaccine could depend on whether one or both—or neither—of these theories is correct.

And while the research on cofactors and genetics goes on, so does the effort to create an AIDS vaccine.

Vaccines traditionally have been made from whole viruses that have either been killed or weakened to the point of harmlessness. Vaccines against polio, measles, smallpox, and yellow fever have all been made this way, and all are very successful. However, most AIDS researchers are reluctant to make an AIDS vaccine from whole virus, either killed or weakened. They don't want to take the remote chance that some live virus will find its way into the vaccine. To get around that problem and still make an effective vaccine, researchers are following other paths.

"One approach is done at the National Cancer Institute, the NCI," said Francis, "where they breed a huge amount of the virus and purify envelope glycoprotein from it. It's kind of a brute-force method, and it's a totally impractical process in terms of getting antigen. It was costing I don't know how many millions of dollars to produce glycoprotein and grow virus. But—he emphasized, "they have done that, and they have inoculated animals and have moved on to chimpanzees. Not with the whole virus, but with a piece of the virus's outer protein coat. This is what's called subunit protein."

A similar approach uses technology at the forefront of

bioengineering. "You take the *gene* for the HIV envelope protein, and insert that gene into some other creature," Francis explained. "It could be the bacterium *E. coli*, for example, which is a common biological factor in genetic engineering. Chiron, the biotech company, is doing this with yeast, and Genentech is using mammalian cells. The advantage of using mammalian cells as a factor for making HIV proteins is that it duplicates the process in other mammalian cells by which the sugars are added on. Is that important?" he said. "We don't know, but it certainly could be."

Because HIV infects helper T cells by plugging into the CD4 receptor, many researchers are focusing on gp120 and gp160, which are HIV surface proteins thought to be involved in the process of binding to the receptor. (That's one reason why the Cambridge BioScience patent on recombinant gp120 may be so lucrative.) This route may be one way around the problem of HIV's high mutability. Another detour may be less technical and more straightforward. Some scientists suggest creating a vaccine that is an "antigen cocktail." Such a "multivalent vaccine" could be made of several proteins that prime the immune system against a constellation of different HIV antigens.

Another approach to an AIDS vaccine is to use the vaccinia virus. This is the route Enzo Paoletti has been following in his development of polyvalent vaccinia-based vaccines. Explained Francis, "You take the vaccinia virus, which is a very large virus, and into it you can insert a large part of the genome of HIV. When the vaccinia replicates in cells, it will not only produce its own proteins, but will produce HIV proteins. The virus acts as a vector, we would say. And you're right. Enzo Paoletti and Bernard Moss have both been the revolutionary people in that process.

"But there's a process that is even beyond the vaccinia vector," he said. "That's to *manufacture proteins,* synthetic polypeptides, in the laboratory. That's what Gordon Dreesman has done. He took the HIV protein p41 and found the part of it that was most likely to be attracted to water." The reason, Francis explained, is that such a water-loving part of the molecule (hydrophilic, scientists would say) is likely to be sticking out of the surface of the virus. That part of p41 would be exposed to the attention of the immune system and thus make a likely candidate for a vaccine antigen. "So Dreesman took a segment out of p41, of either twelve or twenty polypeptides, I forget which, and saw where that water-loving sequence was in the virus. Then he and his people went to their machines in the lab and made the stuff. They then hooked them to a larger molecule that can be recognized by the immune system and began using this compound to immunize small animals, and then chimps."

If this technique works, Dreesman and his colleagues may be able to make a vaccine that primes the immune system against the presence of the p41 AIDS core protein. The immune system doesn't see this antigen until well after a person is infected. However, a p41 vaccine could be given to people who have tested positive for AIDS. It could be the lifesaver for the millions of people already infected with HIV.

Idiotypes and anti-idiotypes may provide a third route to an AIDS vaccine. Ronald Levy and others were using idiotype antibodies in their war against cancer. Dreesman and Ronald Kennedy at the Southwest Foundation for Biomedical Research in San Antonio are trying to make an anti-idiotype AIDS vaccine. They begin by injecting HIV into an experimental animal like a rabbit or chimpanzee. They collect the antibodies which the animal makes in response to the virus. Then the researchers inject the

antibodies into a *second* animal. The second animal makes
antibodies against the injected antibodies. The antibodies
against the antibodies are anti-idiotype antibodies. The
first antibodies could be considered a molecular "mirror"
to the HIV antigen. In the same way, the anti-idiotype
antibodies are molecular "mirrors" of the first antibodies.
Theoretically, therefore, the chemical structure of the
anti-idiotypes should mimic the antigenic structure of the
AIDS virus that was originally injected into the first rabbit.

In other words, if *B* is the mirror image of *A,* and *C* is
the mirror image of *B,* then *A* and *C* should be identical. In
this case *A* is the original antigen on the HIV virus; *B* is the
antibody against *A,* and *C* is the anti-idiotype antibody
against *B.* The whole idea, then, is to use the anti-idiotypes
as a vaccine. Such a vaccine should be completely safe,
since the anti-idiotypes would mimic only the *structure* of
HIV, not its actual genes.

It might also be possible to make anti-idiotypes of the
CD4 receptors on the helper T cells. Such anti-idiotypes
would theoretically tie up the binding sites on the AIDS
virus. In other words, HIV would bind to the anti-idiotype
instead of to the CD4 receptor on the T cells. Such an
anti-idiotype preparation might be effective for people
who are already infected with HIV. Ronald Kennedy, who
leads the anti-idiotype research team at the Southwest
Foundation, has said that he and his colleagues have
already demonstrated in chimps that anti-idiotypes have
potential as a hepatitis B vaccine. A similar approach
might also work for AIDS.

Finally, one could use "old technology" to make an
AIDS vaccine, by resorting to a preparation made from
killed AIDS viruses to trigger the immune system into
action. This is the way the Salk polio vaccine works. Few
AIDS researchers support this route, though. They feel it is
too dangerous to inject people with a vaccine made of dead

HIV. It is always possible, they note, that a few virions could still be alive. And a few HIV are all that's needed to cause AIDS.

Cambridge BioScience is one of many biotech companies hot on the trail of an AIDS vaccine. They're using the recombinant protein approach, relying on their experience with gp120 and a vaccine against feline leukemia virus. During my visit with Richard Thorne at Cambridge Bio-Science's offices in Hopkinton, Massachusetts, he had talked about those efforts. The work began, he confirmed, with their new vaccine against the feline leukemia virus. The FeLV project had involved a lot of molecular biology, and the company's researchers had learned a lot about FeLV, and its different proteins. They had identified the antigens that would be the target of an effective vaccine. The FeLV vaccine that resulted was in preclinical evaluation in 1987, and headed for the marketplace by the end of 1988.

Thorne's comments brought home the difficulty of making a new vaccine. "It's a tremendous undertaking," he said. "Not only do you have to have the right things, but a test system is hard. Everyone looks for super results in the test tube, so you hopefully won't have to go to the 'ultimate system' to do the test. Well, with feline leukemia, it turns out that no one knows what kinds of results in the lab equal real-life protection against the virus. It may be in fact different for each of the three subtypes of the virus. So only one test really counted: Will it protect a cat against the virus?"

The Cambridge BioScience tests were successful. Not only does their FeLV vaccine work, said Thorne, "it works beyond our wildest expectations.

"Now, there's still a lot of work to be done. We must go through a lot of tests, and purification procedures are horrendous for vaccines. I don't know when it will come out. But from the research point of view it is a tremendous project. Maybe it's luck, or good science, or both, but we have done something that no one else has done. Two major companies previously tried to make FeLV vaccines with recombinant methods and failed."

Cambridge BioScience researchers began their creation of the FeLV vaccine with a gene cloned from the feline leukemia virus. They then inserted it into a bacterium called E. Coli, fequently used for genetic engineering. The bacterium expressed the viral gene—it made the protein that it coded for. Next, CB researchers purified the protein.

"Was this a protein from the surface of the virus?" I asked.

Thorne said nothing for a minute; then, cautiously: "I think I can say that's correct, yes."

We were wandering into that territory which the corporate world calls "proprietary information." An effective FeLV vaccine was a veterinary medicine coup. Cambridge BioScience didn't want any competitors stealing its secrets. Especially when one such competitor had tried to make the same vaccine and bombed disastrously.

"You can say that much, then," I said, seeking some sort of confirmation.

"Yes." Another pause. "But I think the most important characteristics are how we purify the protein, and the adjuvants we use. Those are proprietary. We can say that much. And that it's not easy. It was a lot of hard work. You need something to amplify the immune response to a particular antigen. And that's what an adjuvant does. Right now, because of research on AIDS, there is renewed interest in how people and animals actually become immune. There's the cellular and humoral immune responses, of course. But there is also a lot of regulation between the cells of the lymphoid system, and what are called *nonspe-*

cific effectors—macrophages and natural killer cells. And how adjuvants work to amplify the immune response— well, that's an area of very hot pursuit."

Thorne looked slightly apologetic. "Now, I don't think I can give you anything special about this. But basically, the truth is that *no one knows how we become immune*. It all depends on the specific pathogen, on where it enters the body, on what cells see it first. All those things complicate the picture of exactly what immune function kills the infection."

I then asked my first Sixty-Four Dollar Question: Was Cambridge BioScience in fact developing an AIDS vaccine? Thorne nodded yes. "Our approach is to make a vaccine that helps the body develop a state of immunity such that, no matter where the virus enters the body, the immune system can clear it out fast enough to keep it from going and hiding.

"You know," Thorne added in a matter-of-fact tone, "I think HIV is a new virus. A good virus doesn't kill its host. It wants the host to stay alive. The new HTLV virus, HTLV-4 or HIV-2, seems to be a more successful virus, because it doesn't seem to kill its host. That's where HIV would like to be."

"But HIV is an efficient killer of humans," I remarked.

"Oh, I wouldn't call it an efficient killer of people at all," Thorne retorted. "Only in the long term. I think it's very inefficient. It's kind of a blundering virus. It sort of found its little niche, and by accident that happens to be neurons and macrophages and helper T cells. And by accident it causes death. Obviously it's very new in evolutionary terms. A virus that's been around a long time doesn't kill its host."

Thorne made it clear that Cambridge BioScience would not be making an AIDS vaccine on its own. They would do it with a large corporate partner. He felt the company already had a good starting point with their new AIDS antigen test, and with their experience in developing the vaccine for feline leukemia.

What about an animal model for the AIDS vaccine? I asked.

Thorne thought a second. "Chimps are expensive and rare," he said. "So there are several things we can do. For example, we might pursue work with simian AIDS or SAIDS, along with work with HIV. We *can* learn a lot from chimps. At least they can be infected with HIV. In the end we will try doing this in as many in vitro measures as we can. It's possible we would do some chimp experiments if other things are also promising.

"The end point for us, I would say, would not be to stop the disease in chimps *but to see if a vaccine can prevent viremia*. My guess is any vaccine that will stop chimp viremia is a candidate for humans."

What Thorne was talking about was actually quite straightforward. Suppose a chimpanzee is injected with HIV and gets infected. The primate will then have cells circulating in its blood which contain the AIDS virus, and researchers can detect HIV antigen in the blood serum. That state—the presence of viruses in the bloodstream of an infected animal or human—is called viremia. Thorne was saying that, if they came up with a vaccine that could prevent that in chimps, then they would have something very promising.

"Do you think the vaccine you're working on will be as good as the ones that others are working on?"

"What we have now," said Thorne, "is at least as good as what anybody else has, including Genentech. Actually, Genentech tried developing an FeLV vaccine—and got *nowhere*. But they are very good. They have lots of money and very good people.

"But we have data for an AIDS vaccine that are as good

as theirs, or anyone else's. What we're *not* sure of is, What's the appropriate system to begin testing an AIDS vaccine on? We're a small company; we have to be focused. Genentech, or Robert Gallo for that matter, can basically say, 'What can we do, or try?' and then try them all. We can't do that. We have to be picky. On the other hand, that's a discipline that makes us think carefully about what we're doing."

In fact, Thorne said, Cambridge BioScience was already working with one of the biggest medical organizations in the world: the National Institutes of Health. "We're working with them because anybody who wants to get anywhere with HIV *has* to work with NIH. They have so much information."

"In other words," I said, "You're connected with the Robert Gallo group."

There was a long pause. . . . "Yes."

Robert Gallo, of the National Cancer Institute at the National Institutes of Health, was widely credited as one of the codiscoverers of the AIDS virus. Not everyone agreed with that credit—most especially Donald Francis, who was not shy about saying so publicly.

But other controversies swirled about Gallo. Who had first positively identified the virus? Was it Gallo's lab, or that of Luc Montagnier of the Institut Pasteur in France. What should the virus be called? Gallo insisted on HTLV-III, since he was an expert on the HTLV-I and -II viruses, and had thought at first that the AIDS virus was related. Montagnier called it LAV, for "lymphadenopathy-associated virus," since it infected the T cells in lymph glands. Eventually an international committee settled on HIV. Multimillion dollar lawsuits were thrown about in another controversy related to the clash between Gallo's lab and the Insitut Pasteur. This one involved patent priorities for the first generation of AIDS antibody tests.

That controversy finally had to be sorted out by an agreement between the governments of France and the United States. Perhaps most galling to some of his peers, Gallo was a master of public relations. When the U.S. Secretary of Health and Human Services had held a press conference announcing the discovery of the AIDS virus, Gallo had maneuvered himself onto the platform with her. TV anchormen sought him out for network interviews. He punished reporters who wrote inaccurate or (in his eyes) unflattering articles by shunning them. It became a mark of distinction to get a chance to interview him. Robert Gallo became the Carl Sagan of AIDS and immunology.

Yet despite all the controversy that still surrounds him, Gallo remains a powerful figure in AIDS research. His scientific credentials are impeccable. His skill at gaining publicity might be deplored by some of his colleagues, but he is still highly respected as a researcher. Cambridge BioScience might be a small company, but they have a very powerful connection.

"How far away *are* we from an AIDS vaccine, do you think?" I asked.

Thorne shook his head. "It's hard to make that kind of prediction. It would mean you can foresee all the problems. This is a case where there are no existing solutions to some of the very fundamental problems. This is not like a shot to the moon—simple engineering. New knowledge is necessary. How do you predict when new knowledge comes up?

"We can say this: *It's not forever.* A lot of very bright people are working on an AIDS vaccine, and *it will happen.* But it is hard to put a time frame on it." Thorne looked at me. "It may be sooner than a lot of people realize.

"On the other hand, it could be that treatment for AIDS will improve, diagnostics will get better and simpler, and less expensive. Maybe we'll have premarital screening, and hospital screening. If all that cuts down the spread of the virus and the panic, then progress to a vaccine could proceed at a slower pace."

There were also serious problems, Thorne added. "How do you distinguish people who are vaccinated from people who are infected with AIDS? Both will have circulating antibodies to HIV.

"And even if a vaccine works, what are the risks? There is some evidence to suggest that *not vaccinating enough*, getting just one injection without several boosters, can make you *even more* susceptible to a retrovirus." He shook his head. "And gosh, we do not want that! Ooh boy!"

I mentioned the problem of the virus's mutability. "It seems to change its colors a lot," I remarked. "That's another problem for a vaccine."

Thorne nodded. "It's a complicating factor, yes. FeLV is duck soup in this regard, because it doesn't change that much. The fact is, I know of no successful vaccine against a virus like HIV. It's new territory."

I asked Thorne what he thought about AIDS vaccines based on vaccinia virus. "Yeah," he said. "I guess it's been used successfully for some other viruses. But I don't like the idea of putting into a person anything that can grow, if it has AIDS genes linked up to it." He shook his head. "I don't think it will go."

"It won't fly politically?" I asked.

"Right. I know I wouldn't take a vaccine that had vaccinia as the vector."

"You would not?"

"No. I would not. Smallpox was enough. Oh, I think such a vaccine would probably be safe. But if an AIDS vaccine will work with vaccinia, it will work without vaccinia. So why take the risk?"

Of course, some people *are* taking that risk. AIDS is so scary, so devastating, that every possible route to a vaccine is now being seriously considered. For the journey to an AIDS vaccine is proving harder than many first suspected, including Don Francis. When he first wrote the paper in *New England Journal of Medicine,* he was sure that the first go-round in the search for an AIDS vaccine candidate would be successful. He was wrong.

"This virus is very tricky," he told me. "In a sense, it is doing its best to outsmart even our most modern techniques. All of these techniques I've mentioned have been tried in small animals and in chimps, and by and large have either not produced neutralizing antibodies, or the chimpanzees that were challenged with the virus have not been protected."

Despair washed over me, and I shook my head. "So—I don't understand," I said. "What's the point, then? What have we learned?"

"A lot of things," Francis retorted. "For one thing, we now know that we don't have any small animal that parallels humans and chimpanzees. We haven't gotten a good small animal model for the chimpanzee yet. Second, the chimp is . . ." He paused. "Well, we don't understand the chimp model very well, either."

"My understanding is that chimps can be infected with AIDS but they don't show any symptoms," I said.

"I'm not sure that's true," he replied thoughtfully. "I'm not sure that's true. I know, that's what we were saying when we first discovered the chimp model for AIDS. And I was the discoverer. But I can't say that now. Chimps do lose weight, they do get ill. But the thing is, so few animals have been infected, and for such a short period of time, that until five or ten years go by we can't really say that they don't get ill from AIDS."

He leaned forward. "But the truth is, I *don't care if the chimps get AIDS or not.* All I care about is if they get *infected* or not. The initial goal of a vaccine should be to prevent infection. And a chimp is a perfectly good model for that. The problem is, one, we don't know what the ideal infection is, and two, what the ideal *route* of infection is that mirrors real-life situations.

"I mean, what we do now is inject about a thousand tissue-culture-infectious doses into the vein of a chimp. Then we say, 'Is the chimp protected?' Who *knows* what that means in a real-life situation? Most people infected with AIDS are infected by mucus membrane exposure in their genital system. Patricia Fultz did a vaginal exposure of chimpanzee. She showed that you could infect them with HIV very readily just by putting HIV in the vagina. Is that not a better route? Or per rectum, or mucus membrane exposure compared to an intravenous?

"And just what is the minimum dose that will really reflect the small doses you would get in a real-life situation? In transfusions you would get a very small amount of the HIV virus. I fear that we may end up with a vaccine that *overchallenges* the immune system.

"But don't get me wrong. This is typical of any developmental situation. We're using unknowns to scale more unknowns and trying to make sense of it. But that's what you do on the leading edge. You don't sit back and wait for it to be complete."

In March 1987, a few weeks before my visit with Don Francis and about a month after my discussion with Richard Thorne about the Cambridge BioScience AIDS vaccine work, a workshop on the development of an AIDS vaccine took place at the National Institutes of Health in Washington, D.C. Most participants seemed to feel that the first set of clinical trials, called Phase I trials, should involve fewer than twenty volunteers, and that they should not be gay men, drug users, or members of other high-risk groups. Phase II trials should involve forty to 200 people in both high-risk and low-risk groups. The next move, the Phase II trials, would help determine the right dosage for an AIDS vaccine, and the best timing between doses. Phase III trials, finally, would determine how effective a vaccine would actually be at protecting a person from AIDS infection.

That last step will be a difficult one to take. Everyone involved agrees that clinical trials of AIDS vaccines will be long and costly. It can take five years or more for a person infected with human immunodeficiency virus to develop AIDS. So Phase III efficacy tests on humans will have to involve a huge number of volunteers to yield quickly any kind of meaningful statistics.

AIDS vaccine testers find themselves in a situation much like that of physicists looking for evidence of decaying protons. One currrent theory predicts that protons—one of the three subatomic particles that make up all matter—should break apart and decay into other subatomic particles. But such an event would happen only once every million trillion trillion trillion years. Obviously, there's no way a physicist can watch one proton long enough to see if it falls apart. However, the task becomes easier if one watches *a lot* of protons. If one keeps an eye on, say, a million trillion trillion trillion protons at once, there's a statistical likelihood that one of them will decay each year. AIDS vaccine researchers face the same statistical problem with a Phase III test. They want to see evidence of the vaccine's effectiveness, or lack of effectiveness, in some reasonable time period—say, a year or two. But that will mean using tens of thousands of volunteers. Only in this way will there be a likelihood of quickly seeing statistical evidence that a candidate vaccine is working—or not working.

Some of the volunteers in a Phase III test will be in

high-risk groups. Some will not. Some will be given the real vaccine, while others are given a placebo, a fake vaccine that will be probably nothing more than sugar water. Still others may be given injections of a real vaccine, but one for another disease. Only in this way will researchers be able to tell the difference among (1) an immune response against AIDS triggered by the AIDS vaccine, (2) a generalized immune response to *something* being injected into the volunteer, and (3) a psychologically triggered response to the placebo. Responses (2) and (3) would be real immune responses, but would not protect a person against AIDS.

Serious ethical problems could arise with tests of an AIDS vaccine that used placebos as a control. If a vaccine turns out to be effective during a clinical trial, the researchers involved would be morally bound to end the trial and give everyone, including the placebo receivers, the real vaccine. This, of course, might make long-term clinical studies of an AIDS vaccine impossible. This kind of situation developed during the clinical testing of AZT, the drug that seems to prolong the lives of some AIDS victims. Only seven months after a long-term trial began, the survival statistics for some of the volunteers had improved so dramatically that the test was ended and the AZT given to all the participants. It may have destroyed the *long-term* statistical relevance of the test, but it seemed at the time to be the most ethical action to take for the good of all involved. One result of the dramatic results for AZT, and the sudden ending of the clinical trial, was a shortage of the drug. Burroughs Wellcome, which makes AZT, eventually was able to catch up with the demand. The price for an AZT dose is even coming down a bit. However, it's reasonable to assume that the demand for a proven AIDS vaccine will be many times greater than that for AZT.

The legal complications will be at least as great as the ethical ones. What if someone in the trial contracts AIDS, and claims he or she got it from the vaccine? What if someone comes down with AIDS and claims he or she contracted it because he or she *didn't* get the real vaccine? Who will pay for the legal costs? Who will provide insurance to a company making an AIDS vaccine? The swine flu fiasco of the 1970s offers a glimpse of what might come with an AIDS vaccine. The insurance industry refused to give liability coverage to the swine flu vaccine. This was a direct response to huge awards given by courts to people who claimed they were hurt by the side effects of other vaccines. The manufacturers then refused to release the vaccine. Finally, the federal government stepped in, provided insurance for the vaccine, and eventually assumed all liability.

Researchers have identified more than a dozen possible drugs that could help prolong the lives of AIDS patients, or perhaps even halt the disease entirely. Clinical trials continue on them. Meanwhile, the search for vaccine to prevent AIDS infection also continues. Some prototype vaccines are being tested in humans. The first, and most dramatic such test, began in 1987. A French researcher, Daniel Zagury, injected himself with a prototype AIDS vaccine based on genetically engineered vaccinia virus. By the middle of 1988, Zagury had given himself several booster injections with the prototype vaccine. It seemed to be promising. His body was definitely producing antibodies against the AIDS virus. However, the tests of the antibodies were done in test tubes. Zagury had not taken the ultimate step: injecting himself with a tiny sample of AIDS virus to see if his vaccine prevented infection.

Zagury's bold self-experiment came as a shock to many people, including his wife. He hadn't told her ahead of time. I recalled hearing Don Francis quoted on television as saying that he would also be willing to test himself with a prototype AIDS vaccine. Was that still true? I asked.

"Oh, sure. Sure," he replied. "I don't believe that twenty microns of some protein from a dangerous virus are going to do *anything* to you. And besides, I also think that with the situation we have with AIDS, it's worth taking some chances. I don't have any fear at all of a glycoprotein vaccine, like the one Genentech is working on. I *would* ask my wife"—he smiled slightly—"but other than that, no problem.

"Now, I'm not sure such a vaccine would *work*, mind you! But I have no problems giving that to humans. Of course, I'm certainly not going to *challenge* humans the way I would chimpanzees—"

I jumped on his comment. "Ah, that's the question. You're willing to give people the vaccine but not challenge them with the virus to see if it is effective. So how do you know it's effective?"

"What you do," Francis promptly replied, "is go to humans first. No, you can't challenge humans with the virus. But you *can* use humans as a screening gate to *chimpanzees*. You do your initial tests of a prototype vaccine, your Phase I and Phase II tests, on humans. *Then* maybe you'd challenge chimpanzees.

"Now, we can't go out and do efficacy trials on every prototype vaccine. That's expensive and time-consuming. So a human efficacy trial of a vaccine is not something you want to embark on unless you have some reason to believe it will be reasonably efficacious.

"So where am I? Well, I'm in favor of investigating possible vaccines made with proteins from the virus, of early human administration of prototype vaccines if they're made from recombinants—genetically engineered, in other words—and of getting the chimp model worked out."

"Who's working on AIDS vaccines these days?" I asked.

"You've mentioned NCI, Genentech, Chiron. I know that Cambridge BioScience is working on one."

He said, "Repligen is the one that Gallo is working with very closely, but I don't know much about them. The San Antonio group, the Southwest Foundation with Gordon Dreesman and Ronald Kennedy, is doing the synthetic polypeptide work and the idiotype vaccine work. The Institut Pasteur in France is doing some vaccinia work."

"Then there's Paoletti and the vaccinia virus."

"Yeah, Paoletti and Bernie Moss. I think Oncogen's vaccinia-based vaccine is in collaboration with Bernie Moss." Richard Thorne might have thought there was little chance for a vaccinia-based AIDS vaccine, but others obviously disagreed. And they included some big names and big companies.

By the middle of 1988 several different companies had received permission from the FDA to move ahead with Phase I human tests of prototype AIDS vaccines. The first two were Oncogen in Seattle, with its vaccinia-based vaccine, and a tiny operation called MicroGeneSys, headquartered in Connecticut. And much to the surprise and consternation of the large biotech companies, it was MicroGeneSys, the tiny startup, that was first out of the starting block. The progress of its vaccine is illustrative of the difficulties and time-consuming nature of the search for an AIDS vaccine.

The MicroGeneSys prototype is of the subunit type, using the gp160 protein from the surface of HIV. This type and the vaccinia-based vaccines similar to those being developed by Enzo Paoletti seem to be the two leading contenders. The gp160 in the MicroGeneSys vaccine is made in the laboratory with genetic engineering techniques. It does not come from the AIDS virus itself.

The researchers began with a clone of HIV-1 from the

National Institute of Allergy and Infectious Diseases. The clone went to MicroGeneSys. A team led by Malcolm Martin of NIAID, and Mark Cochran and Gale Smith of MicroGeneSys isolated from the HIV clone the gene that codes for the gp160 protein. They removed the gene and placed it into another virus. In this case it was an insect virus called a baculovirus. Researchers then took the genetically engineered insect virus and grew it in a sample of insect cells. The multiplying viruses infected the insect cells in the tissue culture. They did that the way most viruses work, taking over the genetic machinery of the insect cells in the tissue culture and making them produce new viruses instead of more insect cells. In the process, the insect cells produced the various proteins needed to make new viruses. However, these viruses were modified, carrying the gene for the gp160 protein of HIV. So the insect cells also made large quantities of gp160. MicroGeneSys researchers collected the gp160 for their AIDS vaccine work.

The first step to the candidate AIDS vaccine was to test the gp160 on different animals to look for toxic reactions or other side effects. MicroGeneSys used several different kinds of animals, including guinea pigs, rhesus monkeys, and chimpanzees. They found essentially no serious side effects from inoculating the animals with gp160. Next, they sent blood samples from the test animals to Thomas Folks of NIAID. He examined the blood from the test animals, looking for any antibodies to gp160. One of two chimps tested in the first go-round had in fact produced a relatively high level of antibodies to the protein. It was a good sign. It meant that the chimp's immune system was acting to protect the chimp from a protein that is part of the HIV virus's outer envelope. With that, MicroGeneSys applied to the Food and Drug Administration for permission to begin testing its candidate vaccine on humans. Late in 1987 they got permission to move ahead.

These first human tests, coordinated by Clifford Lane of NIAID (one of the leaders in the AIDS vaccine effort), were the Phase I clinical trials. The point of a Phase I trial is not actually to inoculate people with a vaccine and then see if it protects them from the target disease. Rather, researchers have somewhat simpler goals. First, they want to see if the particular vaccine causes any side effects or toxic reactions in the human volunteers. They also want to determine if the people's immune systems react to the vaccine by making antibodies—which is the whole point of a vaccine. Finally, they want to gauge the best dosages for doing that. The Phase I test on MicroGeneSys's vaccine, which has been named VaxSyn (pronounced like "vaccine"), was supposed to last six months. It involved eighty-one volunteers, seventy-five of whom would be gay men. Another six would be men with no personal history of risky sexual behavior—the kind of promiscuous activity frequently associated with AIDS. All would have to test negative for HIV-1, and so must their sexual partners (if any). Finally, all must not have been exposed to the virus in the three months before the trials began.

MicroGeneSys divided the volunteers into four groups, each getting a different dosage of VaxSyn. After four weeks, a third of each group was to get a booster shot of the original dosage of VaxSyn; another third was to get half the original dosage as a booster. The final third of each group would get no booster shot. Three of the six "no risk behavior" men were to be a separate group, and would receive the highest dosages of all.

The remaining eighteen men were the control group. They were to receive no inoculation of VaxSyn. Instead, they would be injected with a harmless sea mollusk protein called KLH. The control goup would give the Micro-GeneSys researchers something to which they could compare the reactions of the volunteers getting the gp160-based AIDS vaccine. The controls would make complement proteins and antibodies to the KLH, but the antibodies to gp160 are different from those to KLH. If the vaccinated volunteers did indeed respond to the VaxSyn prototype vaccine, the differences would be clear. So would any adverse reactions to the vaccine.

While the test proceeded, researchers would be looking for some kind of immune response to the vaccine. Blood from the vaccinated volunteers would be mixed with HIV. If any antibodies to the gp160 had formed, they would presumably latch onto the AIDS virus and keep it from infecting more cells. It would also be possible to remove T cells and macrophages from the blood samples to see if they reacted to HIV in the test tube.

If either or both of these responses took place, the next step would be a Phase II trial. It would last about a year, involve up to 200 volunteers, and further pinpoint toxicity, side effects, and immune response to the vaccine. Finally, if all signs continued to be positive, MicroGeneSys would apply for permission to begin a Phase III test of VaxSyn.

A Phase III trial of any new drug or vaccine is extremely important. The prototype vaccine must by now have shown quite clearly that it primes the immune system to protect the person against the infectious agent. Ordinarily, a Phase III clinical trial begins with the vaccination of the volunteers. Then, some portion of them are "challenged" with the infectious agent that is the target of the vaccine— they are actually given the virus, microbe, or toxin in question. Another group of volunteers gets the vaccine but not the virus. They are the control group.

However, a Phase III trial for an AIDS vaccine could be very dangerous. There is no danger of getting AIDS from the vaccine. That cannot happen with something like VaxSyn. It is made from a protein from HIV's outer coating rather than from the virus's infectious core. But HIV itself is a killer—perhaps 100 percent lethal. Who would volunteer for an AIDS vaccine trial, when it would involve actually being challenged with a dose of HIV?

As Don Francis pointed out to me, these kinds of clinical trials will have to be done differently. One possibility for the MicroGeneSys vaccine might be to use people who are known to be at extremely high risk for AIDS. Perhaps some recovering drug addicts, or gay men who used to be extremely promiscuous, might volunteer for such tests. The choice would be hard. In fact, it is extremely difficult to imagine *anyone* volunteering for a typical Phase III clinical trial for an AIDS vaccine.

At the beginning of 1988, the MicroGeneSys vaccine trial ran into problems. Lane and Anthony Fauci, NIAID's director, had not been able to recruit volunteers into the trial as quickly as they had originally thought. The reasons for the slowness of volunteer recruitment were complex. One factor was probably the possible stigma of developing antibodies to the AIDS virus and being wrongly perceived as having AIDS.

To move things along, Lane and Fauci expanded and modified the MicroGeneSys vaccine trial. First, six medical centers joined the testing program: Johns Hopkins University and the University of Maryland School of Medicine in Baltimore, Baylor College of Medicine in Houston, Marshall University School of Medicine in Vermont, the University of Rochester School of Medicine in New York, and Vanderbilt University in Nashville. This would add seventy-two more people—women as well as men—to the original eighty-one males in the Phase I test. Secondly, one of the two control groups was changed. In the original NIAID trial, one control group would receive a natural blood protein from sea mollusks instead of the candidate AIDS vaccine. In the multicenter study, however, the control group would get injections of hepatitis B vaccine. This would make it possible for researchers to compare the immune system responses of the volunteers directly to two different vaccines that are made using similar genetic engineering techniques.

By the middle of the year, things were looking very good, indeed. About a third of the volunteers in the test had definitely developed antibodies to HIV, according to a preliminary report by Fauci. In several cases, the antibodies developed within two months of the first injection of VaxSyn. The side effects were minimal, mostly fever and some tenderness at the injection site. The Phase I study of the MicroGeneSys AIDS vaccine would be finished by the end of 1988. The volunteers would continue to be medically monitored for another year.

Despite the apparent progress with the MicroGeneSys vaccine, an enormous amount of work remains. "We need to refine our efforts to find an AIDS vaccine," Francis told me. "Can the questions we're asking be refined by better cooperation and coordination of the whole thing? What about a Manhattan-type project? I don't know if that would help or not. If we had the right well-intentioned people, it might all get done.

"Some of us are backing up a little, and saying, 'Let's do this a little more basically. Get the chimpanzee going. And let's not be so biased that the envelope proteins, the gp160 and gp120, are all that exists.' We're using the ultimates in modern technology for the creation of subunit vaccines. Maybe that's not quite so wise."

"Well, of course, there are other proteins involved, too. Others we could use," I said.

"Actually, what I'm talking about is using the whole virus," said Francis.

I was surprised. "The *whole virus?*" Everyone else I had talked with had rejected outright the idea of using HIV itself as a basis of an AIDS vaccine. It was considered simply too dangerous a method for this disease. For polio, sure. For AIDS? No way.

Francis disagreed. "Yes. The whole virus," he said firmly. "I think we can inactivate this virus. I think we can inactivate it very well. We've got information on it, and now we should at least be backing off for insurance and talking about the whole virus, even produced in cell culture and killed, or certainly produced more safely by recombinant DNA technology where you just exclude the reverse transcriptase or something like that. Then you won't get any replicating virus. Now, no companies are really very interested in this," he said. I wasn't surprised. I could hear the screams of the corporate lawyers. "So I'm encouraging them to do a little formal work and move in that direction."

Perhaps his comments were coincidental, perhaps not. But by the end of 1987, one of the living legends of medicine had announced his intention to create a killed-virus AIDS vacccine. The man was Jonas Salk, the inventor of the killed-virus polio vaccine. Through a San Diego–based company named Immune Response Corporation, Salk is taking aim at AIDS with an experimental vaccine made from whole killed HIV-1. It's the same approach he used to defeat polio in the 1950s. He thinks it will work again with AIDS, and without any danger. And in still another departure from medical orthodoxy, Salk's vaccine will not be meant to protect AIDS-free people from infection. Rather, it is meant to be used to treat people who are already infected with the HIV-1 virus. Salk contends that an AIDS vaccine for people already infected makes sense because HIV can take many years to cause the disease.

By early 1988 Salk's initial trial of a killed-AIDS vaccine was in progress. He was helped along by a California state law that gave permission for quick movement of potential AIDS vaccines from the lab to Phase I trials. Salk could be on the right track. At the Fourth International AIDS Conference in June 1988, Salk announced that several human volunteers had responded positively to his prototype killed whole-HIV vaccine.

Oncogen's vaccine was developed by Steve Kosowski and Shiu-Lok Hu in collaboration with Bernard Moss at NIH. Along with Enzo Paoletti, Moss is the leader in the development of vaccinia-based polyvaccines. The three researchers have taken the vaccinia virus and inserted into its genetic code the HIV genes for the gp120 envelope protein and the p25 core protein. Though it had not worked with chimpanzees, the Oncogen researchers had pressed on and gotten the government's approval for initial human tests. It too was in Phase I trials, with volunteers recruited in part through the University of Washington Health Science Center in Seattle, Washington.

Other possible AIDS vaccines are also in the works. The giant San Francisco biotech company Genentech had declined to talk about their AIDS work. But Don Francis had mentioned their work on a subunit AIDS vaccine, as had reports in various medical journals. Ronald Kennedy and Gordon Dreesman at the Southwest Foundation in San Antonio, Texas, are developing an anti-idiotype AIDS vaccine. If it works, it will mimic the three-dimensional structure of gp120 that plugs into the CD4 receptor on helper T cells. That would prevent HIV from infecting the T cells and causing AIDS. Dreesman and Kennedy are also working on a subunit AIDS vaccine based on the p41 envelope protein in HIV.

Every possible route to an AIDS vaccine is therefore being pursued: killed-virus (Salk), subunit (MicroGeneSys, Kennedy and Dreesman, and others), anti-idiotype (Kennedy and Dreesman), and vaccinia-based (Oncogen, Genentech, and others).

The race is on. It is a long one, an ultramarathon. Even the most optimistic researchers admit that an effective AIDS vaccine will not be available until the late 1990s at the earliest. Tens of thousands of men, women, and children in the United States are going to die before a vaccine arrives. The worldwide numbers of deaths will be ten to a hundred times that.

As for a cure—few will hazard a guess as to when *that* medical miracle will finally come to pass.

HIV is so devilishly clever a retrovirus, so immunologically slippery, that AIDS may never be curable. For now, the human body lies helpless before this ultimate threat to the immune system. But for all its horror, AIDS has had at least one positive effect. It has spurred the growth of immunology to a full-out gallop. The science that studies how the body defends itself is growing today like never before. The millions of dollars being poured into AIDS research are having the added effect of boosting immunological research across the spectrum. Our desperate race to understand and defeat the AIDS virus has increased our knowledge of B cells, T cells, and antibodies, of immune receptor complexes, immunological growth factors, and interleukins, of the connections between the immune system and the endocrine system, and the immune system and the nervous system, of stress and immunity, of the effect of the mind on the immune response.

Twenty-five years from now, we may well look back on this time, these years from 1981 through the turn of the millennium, as years not only of great anxiety and despair, but also as years of a great opportunity seized and used, years of incredible potential made real, years that witnessed the greatest medical advances of all time.

For these years we live in now, years of fear and years of AIDS, may in fact be both the worst of times and the best of times in our continuing quest for more effective ways to defend the human body.

Glossary of Terms

active immunity Immunity to diseases which is learned by the immune system through exposure and response to various foreign invaders. It is also called *acquired immunity* and *adaptive immunity*.

adenine One of the four bases in ribonucleic acid (RNA) and deoxyribonucleic acid (DNA), usually abbreviated *A*.

adjuvant One of a number of substances that increase the immune system's antigenic response.

AIDS Abbreviation for *Acquired Immunodeficiency Syndrome*. AIDS is spread by sexual contacts involving the exchange of semen and, less frequently, vaginal secretions, by the exchange of blood in and on shared needles by drug addicts, and, rarely now, the reception of tainted blood in transfusions. AIDS is not spread by any casual social or medical contact, by donating blood to a blood bank, by mosquitoes or other animal vectors, or by kissing, hugging, or caressing. AIDS is characterized by the infection and destruction of various cells by a virus known as HIV. Immune system cells infected and destroyed include helper T cells, B cells, and perhaps even the pluripotent stem cells in bone marrow. AIDS eventually causes the near-total collapse of the immune system. The infected person then contracts various opportunistic infections such as *Kaposi's sarcoma, Pneumocystis carinii pneumonia,* and various fungal infections. AIDS is frequently accompanied by dementia caused by the destruction of various brain cells by HIV. The disease is nearly always fatal, with an average lifespan after full-blown infection of about eighteen months. There is no known cure. No preventative vaccine currently exists.

allele One of two or more different genes containing specific inheritable characteristics, which occupy corresponding positions on paired chromosomes. More than one inheritable characteristic may be present on the same pair of genes or alleles.

alloantigen An antigen present in an individual that stimulates the production of antibodies in other members of the same species but not in that particular individual.

alloantiserum An antiserum containing antibodies to a particular alloantigen.

alpha emitter A version of an element (isotope) which decays radioactively by releasing a helium nucleus, two protons and two neutrons.

amino acid An organic chemical compound which is an essential building block of peptides and proteins.

antibody A protein, one of five major classes of immunoglobulin molecules, produced by the immune system's B cells in response to, and specifically interacting with, a unique foreign substance.

antigen Any substance, either originally external to the body or produced within the body, which the immune system recognizes as being foreign or Not-Self.

antigenic Able to cause the immune system to produce antibodies.

antigenic determinant The specific molecular pattern on an antigen which causes the immune system to identify the compound as Not-Self. The part of the antigen to which an antibody attaches.

autoantigen A substance occurring naturally in the body which the immune system, for some reason, identifies as foreign. When autoantigens trigger an immune response, it is referred to as an *autoimmune response*.

autoimmune disease A disease in which the body's immune system mistakenly attacks the body itself. In autoimmune diseases, the immune system produces antibodies against normal parts of the body, and these antibodies damage the body.

autoimmunity The condition in which the immune system produces antibodies against the body's own tissues.

autosome Any chromosome other than the sex chromosomes.

AZT A drug used to treat some of the symptoms of AIDS in some people with AIDS. Also called *zidovudine*.

B cell One of the major cells of the immune system. B cells, also called B lymphocytes, make antibodies.

B lymphocyte The more scientific name for B cell.

base A chemical substance that combines with hydrogen ions. Four bases make up the essential structure of DNA and RNA.

beta emitter A radioactive isotope that decays by releasing electrons, which used to be called beta particles.

Bordetella pertussis The bacterium which causes pertussis or whooping cough, discovered by the Belgian physician Jules Bordet.

cancer Any one of a very broad group of malignant tumors. Cancer is characterized by the cells' inability to stop growing and dividing. Cancer is invasive and tends to spread to surrounding tissues. Some cancers have environmental causes; others are genetic in origin or in susceptibility; other cancers are caused by viruses.

carcinoma A cancerous tumor which occurs in epithelial tissue —that is, the tissues that form the outer layer of skin and which line body cavities and tubes as mucous membranes.

CD4 receptor A particular three-dimensional molecular structure, which occurs on the surface of certain immune system cells and brain cells, acting as molecular "locks" for specific chemical "keys." It is now known that the AIDS virus, HIV-1, attaches itself to these cells by means of the CD4 receptor. Genetically engineered CD4 is currently being tested as a potential treatment for AIDS.

cellular immune response The immune response characterized by the actions of various types of T cells, also known as *cell-mediated immunity*.

challenge To infect a laboratory animal deliberately with a disease against which the animal has been vaccinated. The purpose is to see if the vaccine is effective—that is, to "challenge" the vaccine.

chimera An organism carrying cell population from two or more different fertilized egg cells; the cell populations may be from different species. In general, a chimera is any biological unit made with pieces from two or more unrelated units. The word comes from Greek mythology. The mythical chimera was a creature which was part lion, part snake, and part goat.

chromosome One of the threadlike structures in the nucleus of a cell that carries genetic information.

class switching The process by which a single B cell or its progeny shifts from the synthesis of one class of immuno-globulin molecule to a second.

clone A group of genetically identical cells or organisms derived from a single common cell or organism through mitosis.

Coccidioides immitis The bacterium whose spores cause the disease known as valley fever.

codon A unit of three adjacent nucleotides along a DNA or RNA molecule that designates (or carries the code, thus the name) for a particular amino acid. Some codons act as stop signals. Different codons in some cases code for the same amino acid. The order of codons along the molecule determines the order of amino acids in a protein chain, and thus the particular protein created.

colony stimulating factor A polypeptide molecule, usually a protein, that triggers and/or stimulates the growth and development of a type of cell.

colorectal cancer A malignant tumor of the large intestine.

complement One of eleven complex enzyme-acting proteins in the blood, which play a role in the humoral immune reaction. In a reaction between antibodies and an antigen, complement kills the antigenic cell. Complement is also involved in violent allergic reactions and in the cell-killing activity of phagocytes.

complementary base pairing The alignment of only certain nucleotides opposite each other in the two strands of DNA. Adenine connects only with thymine (or uracil in RNA), and cytosine only with guanine. Complementary base pairing is the key to DNA's ability to replicate itself after the two strands separate.

contagious Communicable—as a disease which may be transmitted by direct or indirect contact.

cytosine One of the four base chemicals that are fundamental parts of DNA and RNA, usually abbreviated C.

cytotoxic Having a toxic or killing effect on cells.

cytotoxic T cell Another name for killer T cells.

dalton A unit of molecular weight, roughly equal to the weight of a hydrogen atom.

DDC An experimental drug being used to treat some people suffering from AIDS—not a cure for AIDS, but a treatment for some symptoms and opportunistic diseases associated with it.

dimer A compound formed by the union of two molecules of a simpler compound.

DNA Abbreviation for deoxyribonucleic acid, a large molecule found mainly in the chromosomes inside the nucleus of cells, which is the carrier of genetic information. The molecule consists of a sequence of paired bases connected by two outer sugar-phosphate "backbones"; the molecule is twisted into a double helix shape resembling a spiral staircase.

endorphin Any one of several peptides which act in both the central and peripheral nervous systems to reduce pain. Because they produce pharmacologic effects similar to morphine and other opiate drugs, endorphins are called opioid peptides. They include beta-endorphin, met-enkephalin, leu-enkephalin, dynorphin, alpha-neo-endorphin, and many variants.

enzyme A protein molecule whose function is to speed up a biological chemical reaction. Enzymes are generally given names that end in the suffix -*ase*.

eosinophil A nonspecific immune system cell, one of several kinds of leukocytes. Eosinophils constitute 1 to 3 percent of the white blood cells of the body. They increase in number in response to allergies and some infection.

epitope A group of amino acids on the surface of an antigen which causes a specific reaction by an antibody.

erythropoietin A colony-stimulating factor released into the bloodstream, which acts to stimulate and regulate the production of red blood cells.

Escherichia coli A species of bacteria normally found in the intestines, and common in water, milk, and soil. *E. coli* has been used for decades in the laboratory for medical and genetic research. The strains of *E. coli* used in the laboratory are so heavily mutated and modified that they are no longer able to live in nature.

exon That part of a DNA molecule that produces the code for the final messenger RNA.

FeLV *Feline Leukemia Virus,* a retrovirus which causes a form of leukemia in cats.

gene The biologic unit of genetic material and inheritance, a particular nucleic acid sequence within a DNA molecule that occupies a precise location on a chromosome, and which is capable of self-replication by coding for a specific polypeptide chain. In humans and other mammals, genes occur as paired alleles.

gene expression The translation of the genetic information contained in a gene into a protein.

genetic engineering The manipulation of the information content of one organism to alter that organism's characteristics. Genetic engineering is as simple and "old-fashioned" as selective breeding. However, the term now commonly refers to the technology of cutting apart and splicing together different pieces of DNA and RNA to form new DNA and RNA molecules artificially.

genetics The science which studies the principles and mechanisms of heredity, in particular, the means by which traits are passed on from parents to offspring, and the causes of the similarities and differences between related organisms.

genome The complete set of genes in the chromosomes of each cell of a particular organism. The human genome, for example, consists of about 100,000 genes in forty-six chromosomes.

glycoprotein A chemical compound made of a protein and a carbohydrate. The outer envelope or "skin" of some viruses are glycoproteins.

gp120 A glycoprotein component of the human immunodeficiency virus (HIV) which helps form the outer protein envelope of the virus. It is a candidate for several possible AIDS vaccines.

gp160 A glycoprotein product of HIV, which is broken down into gp120 and p41. A genetically engineered version of gp160 is being considered as a possible AIDS vaccine.

granulocyte One of a group of leukocytes which includes eosinophils and neutrophils.

guanine One of the four bases which is a fundamental part of DNA and RNA, usually abbreviated G.

haplotype A group of closely linked genes on a single chromosome that codes for a specific characteristic or function, such as blood type or the immune system's MHC markers.

hapten A nonimmunogenic substance that can combine with an antigen. When it does so, it gives the antigen a new specificity, so that another unique antibody is needed to recognize and attack it.

heavy chain The larger of the two protein chains which comprise an antibody. There are five classes of heavy chains, named alpha, delta, epsilon, gamma, and mu.

helper T cell The subset of T cells which activates or boosts the functioning of B cells. Helper T cells are identified by the presence on their surfaces of a molecular receptor called the CD4 receptor. HIV, the AIDS virus, infects helper T cells and eventually kills them. AIDS is characterized in part by an abnormally low ratio of helper T cells to suppressor T cells.

hematopoiesis The production and development of various blood cells, usually in bone marrow.

Hemophilus influenzae An organism which causes a form of meningitis that often afflicts very young children.

Herpesvirus varicellae The virus which causes chicken pox.

HIV *Human Immunodeficiency Virus,* the cause of AIDS. HIV is a retrovirus which uses reverse transcriptase to insert its genetic code into the genome of infected cells. The length of its incubation period is unknown, but it can apparently exist in human cells for years without becoming active and causing AIDS. HIV is currently known to exist in two major versions called HIV-1 and HIV-2. HIV-1 is responsible for nearly all AIDS cases in the United States and other parts of the world. Only scattered cases of HIV-2 infection have been found outside Africa as of the middle of 1988. HIV's inner core contains at least nine known genes. Its outer protein envelope changes or mutates frequently. Previously known as ARV, HTLV-III, and LAV.

HLA Abbreviation for *Human Leukocyte Antigen* region, the major histocompatibility genetic region in humans, which codes for the markers that identify cells as Self. It is located on human chromosome 6.

horsepox A form of pox which once affected horses. It is now extinct, but is thought by some to be the source of the vaccinia virus used to vaccinate humans against smallpox.

humoral immune response The immune response characterized by the actions of B cells and antibodies.

hybridoma A cell that is made by the fusion of two different cells and which contains genetic material from both. Often, in cancer research and immunology, a hybridoma is a cell artificially produced by fusing together a B cell with a special kind of myeloma cancer cell. The hybridoma has the characteristic of continually growing and reproducing, and also making large quantities of a specific antibody. The resulting antibodies from the hybridoma clone are called monoclonal antibodies.

hydrophilic Having the tendency to attract and hold water.

hypermutation A process of mutation by which nucleotides are scattered randomly through a sequence of gene fragments in the process of combining to create the codes for antibodies.

hypervariable region One of several regions in the variable regions of light and heavy chains, which determine the antigen-binding site of an antibody molecule.

idiotype A unique variable region on an antibody which determines the specific part (epitope) of an antigen that will react with the antibody.

IgA Immunoglobulin A, one of the five major classes of antibodies. It is the predominant antibody found in human bodily secretions such as saliva, tears, nasal mucous, and vaginal secretions.

IgD Immunoglobulin D, the predominant immunoglobulin class found on B cells. It may be involved in B cell growth and maturation. It is found only in trace amounts in human blood serum.

IgE Immunoglobulin E, one of the five major classes of antibodies. It is involved in allergic reactions.

IgG Immunoglobulin G, the predominant class of antibodies found in humans. IgG is the only immunoglobulin that can cross the placenta from mother to fetus, and is responsible for immunological protection of an infant during its first few months after birth.

IgM Immunoglobulin M, present along with IgD on the surface of most B cells. IgM normally exists in clusters of five connected at the bottoms of the Y. It is prominent in the early antibody response to most antigens.

immune response The response of the body's immune system to the presence of foreign substances, including viruses, bacteria, toxins, and other substances such as dust, asbestos fibers, splinters, etc. The immune response is a complex interaction of passive defenses such as skin, and active defenses including the nonspecific immune response, the humoral immune response, and the cellular immune response.

immunity A state of being protected from a disease, particularly an infectious disease.

immunodeficiency A state of weakened immune response.

immunogen Any substance that stimulates the formation of an antibody.

immunoglobulin One of a family of closely related but not identical proteins capable of acting as antibodies. Five major classes of immunoglobulins exist, determined by the presence in the molecule of one of five types of heavy chains. The five classes are *immunoglobulin A* (IgA), *immunoglobulin D* (IgD), *immunoglobulin E* (IgE), *immunoglobulin G* (IgG), *immunoglobulin M* (IgM).

immunology The science which studies the nature and functioning of the immune system.

immunotherapy Treatment of diseases such as cancer by techniques that boost the body's immune system.

in vitro Latin phrase meaning "in glass," referring to a test performed in a laboratory on cells, organs, or isolated tissues in a test tube or petrie dish.

in vivo Latin phrase meaning "in the living body," referring to a test performed on a living organism.

inoculate To inject a microorganism, serums, or toxic materials into the body, done with a needle and syringe, scarification of the skin (scratching with a small needle), or some other method. It is a frequently used method of vaccination.

interferon Any of several proteins produced by infected cells which protect nearby uninfected cells from viral infections. Among other actions, interferon induces the formation of natural killer cells.

interleukin One of several proteins, produced by immune system cells, which stimulate the growth and activation of other immune system cells.

interleukin-1 A polypeptide produced by macrophages, which stimulates the growth and activation of B cells, abbreviated as IL-1. Interleukin 1 is also released by other cells of the immune system, including T cells and B cells, and participates in the activation of various cells and their functions.

interleukin-2 A polypeptide released by helper T cells, which stimulates killer T cells and other T cells and immune system cells, including macrophages, abbreviated IL-2. It was once called T cell growth factor.

interleukin-3 A polypeptide released by T cells, which stimulates certain cells in the bone marrow to begin producing new immune system precursor cells, abbreviated as IL-3.

intron A noncoding section of a gene, which is removed from RNA before the gene is translated into a protein. Found in cells of higher organisms. Bacterial RNA does not have introns.

Kaposi's sarcoma A malignant tumor of blood-vessel tissues in the skin and some internal organs, normally seen only rarely and then primarily in older men of Italian and Jewish origin, and in Africa. A particularly virulent form frequently infects people with AIDS.

killer T cell A subset of T cells which directly kills invading microorganisms. Also called cytotoxic T cells. Killer T cells are antigen-specific, and can kill repetitively. They contain on their surfaces receptors for interleukin 2, and are activated by reacting with IL-2.

leukocyte Any of several kinds of immune system cells that are nonspecific in the kinds of foreign substances they attack. Leukocytes act as scavengers, surrounding, eating, and digesting foreign substances.

leukotriene Any of a class of chemical compounds involved in the inflammatory reaction to foreign substances.

light chain The smaller of the two protein chains that comprise an antibody molecule.

locus In genetics, the site of a gene on a chromosome.

lymph A fluid found in lymphatic vessels, usually clear, transparent, and colorless. Lymph is formed in the spaces between all body tissues, and drains from there through the lymphatic system into the bloodstream. Lymph contains many different proteins, salts, organic substances, and water. Cells present in lymph include various immune system lymphocytes.

lymphatic system The system of ducts and tissues which convey the fluid called lymph from the body's tissues to the bloodstream. The lymphatic system includes lymph capillaries, lymph nodes, lymph vessels, and lymph ducts. It is a significant part of the immune system, since many immune system cells reside in lymph nodes, where they detect and attack antigen-bearing organisms and particles which are being carried in the lymph.

lymphocyte Any of several kinds of lymph cells. The term usually refers to B lymphocytes or B cells, and T lymphocytes or T cells.

lymphokines The protein products of lymphocytes which act as the messenger chemicals of the immune system, responsible for the multiple effects of the immune reaction.

macromolecule An extremely large molecule—for example, a protein.

macrophage Nonspecific immune system cells with the ability to eat microscopic particles and organisms which enter the body. After digesting the foreign object, the macrophage returns some of the partly digested antigen to its surface, where the antigen can be detected by helper T cells. Macrophages also carry on their surfaces MHC class I antigens. A helper T cell must recognize and react with both antigens for it to be activated.

metastasize To spread from one location in the body to another, especially in reference to the spread of cancerous cells.

MHC Abbreviation for *major histocompatibility complex;* the collection of genes in an organism's genetic code which codes for the Self-marker proteins. Some MHC proteins or antigens, appear on the surfaces of all the body's cells, and mark them as belonging to the body and not foreign. Other MHC antigens appear only on the surfaces of certain immune system cells, and restrict the action of T cells. The human MHC region is called the HLA region and is found on chromosome 6.

MHC restriction The limitation of the action of T cells by the presence on other immune cells of certain molecules produced by the MHC region.

MHC-encoded protein The Self-marker proteins encoded by the genes of the major histocompatibility complex.

mitosis A type of cell division that takes place in somatic cells, which results in two genetically identical daughter cells containing the number of chromosome pairs for that species. Mitosis is the process by which the body makes new cells for both growth and for repair of injured tissue.

mixed lymphocyte response The mutual immune response reaction, which occurs when lymphocytes from two different organisms are mixed together. The T cells of each organism respond to the MHC antigens of the other by growing and becoming activated.

monoclonal antibodies Identical copies of antibody produced by hybridomas, the fused product of a B cell and a myeloma cancer cell.

monocyte One of several phagocytes or leukocytes, character-ized by being very large, with much more protoplasm than other leukocytes. A monocyte participates in the nonspecific immune response, and is abundantly found at the sites of delayed allergic reactions.

mRNA Abbreviation for *messenger RNA,* the RNA which carries the information first contained in a gene's DNA to a ribosome, where it is translated into a protein.

mutagenic Capable of causing genetic mutations.

mutation A change in a gene potentially capable of being transmitted to the organism's offspring.

myasthenia gravis An autoimmune disease characterized by great muscular weakness and progressive fatigue. The im-mediate cause is a lack of a certain neurotransmitter chemical, resulting in the nerve impulses failing to induce normal muscular contraction. The lack of the neuro-transmitter is caused by an autoimmune reaction.

natural immunity A more or less permanent immunity to dis-ease with which a person is born, due in part to the natural presence of various immune system cells, as well as diet, metabolism, and/or genetically adaptive features.

natural killer cells A type of nonspecific immune system cell which acts to recognize and rapidly kill several kinds of cancerous and bacterially infected cells, often abbreviated as NK cells. NK cells are being used experimentally as treatments for various kinds of cancers.

Neisseria gonorrhoeae The bacteria which causes gonorrhea.

neoplasm Any abnormal growth of new tissue, either benign or malignant, also called a *tumor.*

neutropenia An unusually small number of neutrophil cells in the blood.

neutrophil One of the class of nonspecific immune system cells that act to attack and eliminate foreign invaders before the activation of antibody formation. Neutrophils, along with macrophages and other nonspecific immune cells, have the same immediate cellular ancestor separate from the immediate precursor cells for B and T cells. All three precursors derive from the pluripotent stem cell in bone marrow.

nonspecific immune response The immune response carried out by immune cells such as macrophages and phagocytes. It involves the activation of the complement system and the inflammatory response of cells and tissues to foreign organisms and particles. It does not involve the stimulation of antibodies.

nucleotide A chemical compound consisting of a base, sugar, and phosphate. DNA and RNA look like twisted ladders, and the nucleotide is a structural unit. The sugar and phosphate make a segment of the outer rail, and the base is part of the step or rung.

oncogene A gene which in some way codes for a susceptibility to a cancer.

p18 A glycoprotein component of HIV, which helps form the core surrounding the viral RNA and reverse transcriptase.

p24 One of the glycoprotein components of HIV, which helps form the core of the virus, enclosing the RNA.

p41 A glycoprotein component of HIV, which along with gp120 forms the outer coat of the virus.

peptide A compound made of two or more amino acids, and intermediate in weight between amino acids and proteins.

peptide T A peptide about eight amino acids long, which is a key part of the CD4 receptor on helper T cells. Artificially made peptide T is being tested as a possible treatment of AIDS.

pertussis Whooping cough, an infectious disease caused by the bacteria *Bordetella pertussis,* characterized by inflammation of mucous membranes, followed by a distinctive wracking cough and ending in a whooping intake of breath.

phagocyte A nonspecific immune system cell that surrounds and digests microorganisms and cell debris.

pluripotent stem cell The cells in the bone marrow that are the parents of blood and immune system cells.

Pneumocystis carinii pneumonia A form of pneumonia very common in people with AIDS.

polypeptide A large peptide molecule, often used to refer to a protein.

prostaglandin Any of a class of chemical compounds that are involved in the body's inflammatory response to foreign substances.

protein A class of long chainlike molecules made of hundreds of amino acids.

receptor A large molecular complex on the surface of a cell, which interacts with an external chemical compound to change the function of the cell. The receptor acts like a lock that opens to a specific chemical key. On the cells of the immune system, the key for the receptor lock is usually a lymphokine or an antigen.

recombinant DNA A chimeric DNA molecule made by splicing different DNA fragments together, using genetic engineering technology.

retrovirus A virus that uses RNA instead of DNA as the carrier of its genetic information.

reverse transcriptase An enzyme that makes DNA from RNA, and converts the DNA copy into a double-stranded form, which can be inserted into the genome of the infected cell. It is essential to the functioning of retroviruses, including HIV, the AIDS virus.

rheumatoid arthritis An autoimmune disease characterized by inflammatory changes in the joints and related structures that results in crippling deformities. A very strong genetic tendency has recently been proved, and the location of the genes has been fairly well determined.

ribavarin An experimental AIDS drug being tested to determine its effectiveness against certain opportunistic illnesses in people with AIDS.

ribosome A large ball-like structure inside a cell which acts as a workbench for the construction of proteins. Ribosomes are made of a special kind of RNA called ribosomal RNA and about fifty specialized proteins.

RNA Abbreviation for ribonucleic acid. It is a long, thin, chainlike molecule usually found as a single chain. RNA is similar in structure and composition to DNA. It is made of nucleotides using three of the four bases found in DNA. RNA uses the base uracil instead of thymine and the sugar ribose instead of deoxyribose. RNA controls the creation of proteins in all living cells, and takes the place of DNA in some viruses. RNA comes in several different forms.

sarcoma A cancer arising from connective tissue such as muscle or bone, which may affect the bones, bladder, kidneys, liver, lungs, and spleen.

sequence An arrangement or order of a series of items—in genetics, the arrangement of nucleotides in a DNA or RNA molecule.

smallpox A highly contagious disease, which was caused by the variola virus. It was characterized by chills, headache, and the appearance of serious pustules and eruptions on the skin. Smallpox is considered to have been completely eradicated. The virus is extinct in the wild.

somatic Pertaining to nonreproductive cells or tissues.

specific immune response An immune response that occurs in the presence of a specific antigen or disease, and which involves all changes associated with antigen contact by the immune system.

subunit vaccine A vaccine consisting of a part of a viral protein, often a piece of the outer envelope that does not change as the virus mutates. Subunit vaccines are usually made using genetic engineering techniques.

suppressor T cell A subset of T cells that act to slow down and stop the cellular immune response of T cells and their associated lymphokines. AIDS is characterized by an abnormally high ratio of suppressor T cells to helper T cells.

T cell Any of several kinds of immune system cells which mature in the thymus gland, and which participate in the functions of the cellular immune response, also known as T lymphocyte.

T lymphocyte The more scientific name for T cell.

thymine One of the four bases which form DNA, usually abbreviated as T. It is not found in RNA, which uses uracil.

thymocyte An immature T cell, which has migrated from bone marrow to the thymus.

thymus An organ located behind the breastbone and above the heart, in which immature T cells called thymocytes differentiate into their different subsets and reach maturity. The thymus is essential to the development of the immune response in newborns. It is about 13 grams in weight at birth, grows rapidly the first two years, and then more slowly, reaching a maximum weight of about 30 grams at puberty. The thymus then slowly shrinks and finally disappears during adulthood.

toxin A poisonous substance of animal or plant orgin.

toxoid A toxin that has been treated to destroy its toxicity, but which still is capable of stimulating the formation of antibodies.

tRNA Abbreviation for transfer RNA, a small form of RNA that positions amino acids in the correct order during protein synthesis in the ribosome. tRNA uses information from mRNA to position the amino acids correctly, a process which takes place before the amino acids are actually joined together.

tumor necrosis factor A polypeptide produced by macrophages, which activates a variety of immune system responses. Abbreviated as TNF, it was originally identified as a chemical which can kill cancerous cells. TNF is now known to influence the functioning of cells such as T cells, B cells, connective-tissue cells, and bone marrow cells that produce blood cells. TNF is being actively investigated as a potential cancer-fighting or cancer-curing compound.

uracil One of the four bases that forms RNA, usually abbreviated *U*. It is not found in DNA, which uses the base thymine.

vaccination Inoculation with a vaccine to establish resistance to a specific infectious disease.

vaccine A liquid suspension of infectious agents, or some part of them, given for the purpose of creating resistance to an infectious disease.

vaccinia A virus of the poxvirus family, used as a vaccine against smallpox. Vaccinia is now being used in the creation of genetically engineered vaccines, or polyvaccines, against many diseases at once.

variola The virus which causes smallpox. Smallpox is considered to have been totally eradicated, and the virus is extinct in the wild. Only small amounts of variola still exist in a few laboratories.

VaxSyn An experimental AIDS vaccine based on a genetically engineered version of the HIV glycoprotein gp160.

zidovudine Another name for AZT, a drug which is used to alleviate the symptoms of some people with AIDS.

Index

237

Joel Davis is a free-lance science writer. His articles and news reports have appeared in nearly every major popular science magazine in America, including *OMNI, Science Digest,* and *Science News.* He is the author of two previous popular science books, *Endorphins: New Waves in Brain Chemistry* and *Flyby: The Interplanetary Odyssey of Voyager II,* and coauthor of *Mirror Matter: Pioneering Antimatter Physics.* He lives in Olympia, Washington.